武汉大学规划教材建设项目资助出版

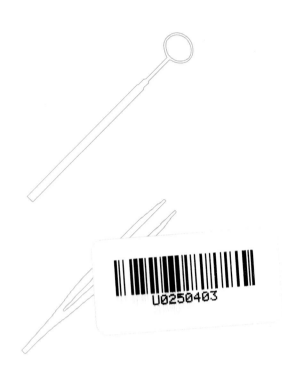

口腔医学专业英语

主编　边专

English in Stomatology

第二版

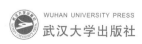

WUHAN UNIVERSITY PRESS

武汉大学出版社

图书在版编目(CIP)数据

口腔医学专业英语 / 边专主编. -- 2 版. -- 武汉 : 武汉大学出版社,
2025. 1. -- ISBN 978-7-307-24736-9

Ⅰ. R78
中国国家版本馆 CIP 数据核字第 2024A5W890 号

责任编辑:鲍 玲　　　责任校对:汪欣怡　　　装帧设计:马 佳

出版发行:**武汉大学出版社**　(430072　武昌　珞珈山)
(电子邮箱:cbs22@ whu.edu.cn 网址:www.wdp.com.cn)
印刷:武汉中科兴业印务有限公司
开本:787×1092　1/16　印张:15.5　字数:310 千字　插页:2
版次:2006 年 8 月第 1 版　　2025 年 1 月第 2 版
　　2025 年 1 月第 2 版第 1 次印刷
ISBN 978-7-307-24736-9　　定价:69.00 元

编 委 会

前　言

　　全球一体化的深入发展对口腔医学专业人才提出了更高的要求。专业英语是国际交流的重要媒介，是新知识传播和新技术革新的支撑。专业英语的熟练掌握也增强了职业胜任力。伴随着新一轮科技革命的兴起，口腔医学各个领域的知识与技术也得到了较大发展，因此，我们对第一版《口腔医学专业英语》进行了更新与修订。

　　本教材保留了第一版教材的结构。第一部分是情景对话，根据目前国内口腔接诊的习惯与现状对这一部分进行了修订，涉及不同诊疗场景与人物，如预约口腔检查、临床诊疗等；第二部分对口腔专业知识进行了更新，使其更适应于阅读者的英语水平与专业能力，同时图文并茂，增加了可读性和趣味性；第三部分为词汇表。经过修订后的第二版教材内容更加精简，既有对上版教材的传承，又有更新的内容，使其更适合本科生、研究生以及口腔从业者使用。本教材不仅可以帮助本科生为今后的学习打好基础、培育国际视野、提升文化自信，而且可以帮助学习者深化职业理想与职业道德教育，提升综合素养，以应对不同文化背景的交流。

　　第二版我们邀请了许多中青年学者和专家参与了修订和审稿，感谢老师们的辛勤付出。

　　由于时间受限以及编者水平有限，虽然我们尽力为读者呈现一本实用性与专业性并存的教材，但难免有疏漏，敬请广大读者批评和指正。有疑问可以直接联系主编或副主编，边专：bianzhuan@ whu.edu.cn；郭继华：jihuaguo@ whu.edu.cn；尹伟：kq000933@ whu.edu.cn。

边专

武汉大学口腔医学院

2024 年 10 月

Contents

001   **Part 1   Conversation**
003   Unit 1   Conversation in Dental Clinics

019   **Part 2   Clinical Presentations**
021   Unit 2   The 'Normal' Dentitions
026   Unit 3   Tooth Eruption and Exfoliation
032   Unit 4   Properties of Tooth Tissue
041   Unit 5   Caries
048   Unit 6   Caries in Deciduous Teeth
055   Unit 7   Tooth Isolation
063   Unit 8   Cavity Preparation for Plastic Tooth Restorations
069   Unit 9   Choice of Plastic Restorative Materials
074   Unit 10   Pulp Therapy (Deciduous Teeth)
080   Unit 11   Pulp Removal and Pulp Canal Obturation
                        (Permanent Teeth)
088   Unit 12   Periodontium
097   Unit 13   Dental Plaque, Calculus and Diseases of the
                        Gingivae and Periodontium

Contents

106   Unit 14   Caries Prevention and Plaque Reduction

117   Unit 15   Prevention of Periodontal Disease

124   Unit 16   Crowns and Bridges

142   Unit 17   Partial Dentures and Complete Dentures

155   Unit 18   Extraction of Teeth

162   Unit 19   Biopsy

169   Unit 20   Benign Swellings in the Oral Cavity

176   Unit 21   Odontogenic Tumours and Tumour-like Lesions

184   Unit 22   Implant-retained Options

191   Unit 23   Reading and Reporting Radiographs

198   Unit 24   Orthodontic Assessment

205   Unit 25   Orthodontic Appliances

217   **Part 3   Index**

219   Vocabulary

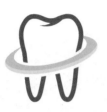

Part 1
Conversation

Unit 1 ▶ Conversation in Dental Clinics

▤ Making an Appointment I

Mr. Miller: I'd like to schedule an appointment with a dentist.

Dental Assistant: Of course. Are you looking for a routine check-up, or is there a specific issue you're concerned about?

Mr. Miller: Yes, I'm having trouble with a tooth that's very painful when I chew.

Dental Assistant: Can I get your name and contact number, please? Do you have basic medical insurance?

Mr. Miller: My name is Berg, and my phone number is 12714566168. I don't have basic medical insurance.

Dental Assistant: We should examine that tooth as soon as possible to figure out what's causing the pain. If you're available, we have an opening tomorrow afternoon at 3 p.m.

Mr. Miller: That's very considerate of you. I'll take that appointment. One more thing, what will you do during the appointment, and how much will it cost?

Dental Assistant: Doctor Wu will examine the tooth and likely take some X-rays. Once we know what's going on, we'll discuss your treatment options with you. The initial consultation, including the X-rays, will cost 60 yuan.

▤ Making an Appointment II

Mrs. Carroll: Hello, I'm Rose Carroll. Could I schedule a dental check-up for next Monday morning?

Dental Assistant: I'm sorry, we're fully booked that day. How about Tuesday morning at

10 a. m. instead?

Mrs. Carroll: That sounds good. But if there's a cancellation on Monday morning, could you please contact me? My phone number is 12836745166.

Dental Assistant: No problem, I'll make a note of that. Have you been to our clinic before? If you're already a patient, could I have your patient record number?

Mrs. Carroll: No, I'm a new patient, but I know where your clinic is because one of my colleagues, Mrs. Liu, recommended your office.

Dental Assistant: Great! I look forward to seeing you on Tuesday.

🗒 Examination I

Dr. Yu: Good afternoon, Mr. Davis. I'm Dr. Yu, and I'll be conducting an examination of your teeth and mouth. Are you experiencing any specific issues with your teeth or gums?

Mr. Davis: Good afternoon, Dr. Yu. I'm not in pain, but it's been a long time since my last check-up, and I'm feeling a bit anxious.

Dr. Yu: I completely understand, and I'll make sure to keep you as comfortable as possible. How long has it been since your last dental visit?

Mr. Davis: I believe my last visit was about two and a half years ago, but I'm not entirely sure.

Dr. Yu: How often do you typically visit the dentist?

Mr. Davis: As I mentioned, I'm nervous about dental visits, and my busy schedule doesn't help, so I don't go regularly. I usually only go for a check-up if I feel it's been too long or if I notice any issues with my teeth.

Dr. Yu: I see. Since this is your first visit to our clinic, I'll need you to fill out a health questionnaire. It includes a few important questions, and I'd appreciate it if you could complete it before we proceed with the examination.

(*During the oral examination*)

Dr. Yu: Mr. Davis, you'll feel me using an instrument to check for cavities and to assess the condition of any existing fillings and crowns. I'll also examine your gums, which might cause a bit of discomfort as I check around and between your teeth.

Dr. Yu: I've finished the examination. I'd like to take some X-rays to check for any issues between your teeth and beneath the gums.

Examination II

Dr. Cui: Good morning, Mr. Smith. How are you today? What seems to be the problem?

Mr. Smith: Good morning, Dr. Cui. I'm doing well, except for this tooth on the upper right side that's been hurting on and off for the past few weeks.

Dr. Cui: I see. When was your last dental visit? Do you remember where you saw your last dentist?

Mr. Smith: I usually try to visit a dentist at least once a year, but it can be challenging because I travel frequently for work. I think my last visit was about six months ago when I was in Guangzhou.

Dr. Cui: Did you receive any treatment during that visit?

Mr. Smith: Yes, I had a cavity in one of my upper right teeth, and the dentist filled it.

Dr. Cui: I noticed from your medical history that you have high blood pressure. Are you currently under the care of a doctor or hospital? Besides the medications you mentioned, have you been advised to take any other measures to control your blood pressure?

Mr. Smith: Yes, my blood pressure is monitored regularly, and my doctor advised me to eat healthier and avoid very salty foods.

Dr. Cui: Alright. Let's take a look inside your mouth now, and I'll check your teeth and gums.

Examination III

Miss Berney: Good afternoon, Dr. Chen. I'm here for a dental check-up, but I'm concerned about my wisdom teeth. I've been feeling some pain on the lower right side, and my friends think it might be my wisdom tooth.

Dr. Chen: I understand. Before we check your wisdom teeth, I need to get a sense of your overall health. Here's a standard medical questionnaire—please take your time to answer all the questions.

(*After completing the questionnaire*)

Dr. Chen: I see that you're generally fit and healthy. Let's proceed with the oral examination.

(*During the examination*)

Dr. Chen: The condition of your teeth and gums looks good overall. I can see that your lower right wisdom tooth is erupting, and the gums around it are a bit swollen. However, I don't see any other wisdom teeth. I'd recommend taking a panoramic X-ray of your jaws to determine the number and positions of all your wisdom teeth.

Miss Berney: Yes, I'll have the X-ray taken, but could you tell me if it's going to hurt?

Dr. Chen: No, Miss Berney. This type of X-ray is usually painless, but you'll need to stay very still while it's being taken.

📇 Presentation of Treatment Plan I

Dr. Shen: Mrs. Brown, I've completed the examination and developed the X-ray films. Let me review your teeth and gums with the X-rays.

Mrs. Brown: Okay, doctor.

Dr. Shen: I've identified a couple of cavities that need attention. One of them appears to be quite deep and may affect the nerve inside the tooth. There's also a broken old filling in one of your upper front teeth that needs to be replaced. Before we proceed with the fillings, you'll need to see the hygienist for a thorough cleaning of your teeth and gums.

Mrs. Brown: Is the cleaning really necessary? I don't feel any pain in my gums.

Dr. Shen: Even if you're not experiencing pain, I've noticed that some areas of your gums are red and swollen, which usually indicates a need for better cleaning. Additionally, your teeth have some staining, likely from tea, and there are multiple deposits of tartar that need to be addressed.

Mrs. Brown: Can I postpone the cleaning and have the fillings done first?

Dr. Shen: It's possible, but I would advise against it. Cleaning your teeth and gums first will improve your oral health and make the filling process smoother and more effective.

Mrs. Brown: I have two other questions. What type of material will you use to replace the broken filling in my upper front tooth? I want it to look natural. Also, if one of the cavities is very deep and affects the nerve, does that mean the tooth will need to be extracted?

Dr. Shen: I'll use a tooth-colored material for the new filling, so it will blend seamlessly with your natural tooth. If the nerve is affected, we can still save the tooth with a root canal treatment, but a crown will be needed afterward to protect it. Extraction would only be considered if the tooth cannot be saved.

Mrs. Brown: Thank you for answering all my questions, doctor.

Presentation of Treatment Plan II

Dr. Qin: Mr. Allen, based on my examination, it's clear that your dental health requires significant treatment to address the issues in your mouth.

Mr. Allen: Yes, I've been aware that my teeth are in poor condition for some time. Can you detail the treatment needed? I'd like to save as many teeth as possible.

Dr. Qin: First, you'll need to see our hygienist to improve your oral hygiene and undergo several sessions of cleaning for your teeth and gums. Four of your back teeth are beyond saving and should be extracted as soon as possible. After that, we'll restore the cavities in your remaining teeth. Two teeth with deep decay will likely require root canal treatment and crowns. Additionally, we'll need to discuss options to replace the missing teeth.

Mr. Allen: That seems like quite a lot of work. Could you explain the options for replacing the missing teeth?

Dr. Qin: To replace the missing teeth, we can consider dentures, bridges, or implants. I have some informational leaflets that explain each option in detail. Please take one home to review, and we can discuss any questions you have at your next appointment.

Mr. Allen: Thank you. Given the extensive treatment needed, I'm concerned about the cost. Can you provide an estimate and explain the payment arrangements?

Dr. Qin: I understand your concerns. I'll provide you with a detailed cost estimate for the treatment. For payment, you can pay as you go. We accept cash, major credit cards, and cheques.

Treatment—Simple Operative Procedures

Dr. Nu: Good morning, Nisha. How are you today?

Nisha: I'm fine, thank you.

Dr. Nu: Did you go to school this morning?

Nisha: Yes, but I had to leave early to come here. What will you be doing today?

Dr. Nu: Last week, I noticed a small cavity in one of your upper back teeth. Today, I'll clean it and place a small filling to prevent it from getting worse.

Nisha: Will it hurt?

Dr. Nu: I'll numb the area with a special gel and a small injection. Once the area is numb, you shouldn't feel any pain. Is that okay with you?

Nisha: I suppose so. But I'd like to hold my mother's hand.

Dr. Nu: Of course. Mrs. Hua, could you hold Nisha's hand, please?

Mrs. Hua: Certainly, doctor.

Dr. Nu: Nisha, I'm going to apply some numbing gel to your gums next to the tooth. This will make your gums numb. Try to keep your mouth open and avoid touching the area with your tongue, as the gel might taste a bit strange.

(*After* 1 *to* 2 *minutes*)

Dr. Nu: I'm going to numb the tooth further now. Please stay still. You shouldn't feel anything. You can squeeze your mother's hand if you need to.

(*After the injection*)

Dr. Nu: Rinse your mouth, and we'll wait a few minutes for the numbness to take effect.

(*After* 3 *to* 4 *minutes*)

Dr. Nu: Does your cheek feel a bit numb and swollen?

Nisha: Yes, it feels really strange. Do I look swollen?

Dr. Nu: No, you look normal. The sensation will pass in about 2 hours. Mrs. Hua, please remind Nisha not to bite her cheek accidentally.

Dr. Nu: I'm going to start cleaning out the cavity now. You might hear some noise and feel vibrations. There will be water splashing in your mouth, and my nurse will use a suction tip to remove it. Keep your mouth open and still, and it will be over quickly.

(*After cavity preparation*)

Dr. Nu: Great job, Nisha! I've finished cleaning the cavity. Now, I'll fill it to prevent food from getting inside.

Mrs. Hua: Excuse me, Doctor. What type of filling will you use? I'd prefer something durable that won't fall out easily.

Dr. Nu: I'll use a white resin filling. It blends well with your tooth color and is quite durable.

Mrs. Hua: Thank you for the information.

Dr. Nu: Nisha, I'm going to fill the cavity now. You may feel some pressure as I place the material. You won't feel any pain, but keep your mouth open so the cavity remains dry. My nurse will use a salivary ejector to keep your mouth dry.

(*After placing the restoration*)

Dr. Nu: Gently close your back teeth together. I've placed a small red film between your teeth to check your bite. Please close your teeth gently again and slowly grind them together.

(*After checking the occlusion and articulation*)

Dr. Nu: All done, Nisha. You can rinse your mouth, but be careful as your face is still numb and you might spill some water.

Dr. Nu: Mrs. Hua, please make sure Nisha avoids biting his cheek while numb. she can eat later this evening, around 7, when the numbness will have worn off. For now, offer soft foods and remind her to chew on the other side to avoid putting pressure on the new filling.

Mrs. Hua: I'll follow your advice. When should I bring her back? I remember you mentioned other teeth needing treatment.

Dr. Nu: Please see the receptionist on your way out to schedule Nisha's next appointment. We'll need to clean and seal some of the back teeth to prevent future decay.

Mrs. Hua: That sounds good. I'll arrange the appointment with the receptionist. Thank you, doctor.

Treatment—Scaling and Oral Hygiene Instructions

Dr. Su: Good morning, Mrs. Carter. How are you this morning?

Mrs. Carter: I'm fine, thank you. What are you going to do today?

Dr. Su: I'm going to clean your teeth and gums, and then I'll go over some oral hygiene instructions so you can keep your teeth clean at home.

Mrs. Carter: What exactly are you going to do when you clean my teeth? Is it going to hurt a lot?

Dr. Su: First, I'll need to remove all the tartar deposits on your teeth. These are usually found around the gum line but can also be located underneath the gums in the gum pockets. I'll use an ultrasonic scaler, which produces vibrations, a lot of noise, and water. I'll also use some hand instruments to clean the areas that are more difficult to reach with the ultrasonic scaler. After that, your teeth will be polished. Since your teeth have had a lot of tartar deposits for a long time, your gums are very inflamed. This means you'll experience some discomfort while I'm scaling your teeth, and you'll notice some bleeding from your gums as I clean around your mouth. This is due to the inflamed condition of your gums.

Mrs. Carter: Okay, doctor, but please be gentle.

(*After completing the scaling*)

Dr. Su: Excellent, Mrs. Carter. I've finished the cleaning for this session. Before you go, I think it's important for me to explain some techniques to keep your teeth and gums healthy. Let's start with tooth brushing. What kind of toothbrush and toothpaste do you use, and how often do you change your toothbrush?

Mrs. Carter: I don't use a particular brand of toothbrush. I usually pick the cheapest and hardest one on the supermarket shelf. I change the toothbrush when the bristles look very worn out, usually every 5 or 6 months. As for toothpaste, I use a smoker's toothpaste to help get rid of stains, but it doesn't seem very effective.

Dr. Su: I'd recommend using a major brand of toothbrush, not the cheapest or hardest one. A major brand toothbrush is usually of better quality, though it might be slightly more expensive. However, a better quality toothbrush is better for keeping your teeth and gums healthy. A hard toothbrush could potentially damage your teeth and gums over time. You should brush your teeth twice a day and change your toothbrush every 2 to 3 months. As for smoker's toothpaste, it's usually more abrasive and could harm your teeth. I'd suggest using a normal toothpaste containing fluoride. I'll show you a good technique to clean your teeth on this model, and I'll give you a leaflet about the tooth brushing technique to take home. Do you use dental floss?

Mrs. Carter: Thank you for all your advice and instructions. I'll try to follow your recommendations. I've tried using dental floss before, but I've always found it very tricky to use.

Dr. Su: Yes, most patients find dental floss difficult to use at first and often give up. However, if you persevere, you'll be able to use it without any problems. Dental floss is a simple way to keep the areas between your teeth and underneath the gums clean. Normal tooth brushing isn't enough to clean these areas effectively. Let me show you how to floss using this model, and then you can try it in front of a mirror.

(After practicing tooth brushing and flossing)

Mrs. Carter: Dr. Su, thank you for your patience and time. I'm a bit worried about the blood from my gums, and they also feel slightly sore.

Dr. Su: At this stage, it's normal for your gums to bleed easily, and for your teeth and gums to feel uncomfortable. However, if you keep them clean as I've shown you, the inflammation around your gums will improve, and you'll notice the bleeding and discomfort will lessen after a short time.

🗒 Treatment—Root Canal Treatment

Dr. Bian: Good morning, Mr. Wright. How are you today?

Mr. Wright: I'm fine, thank you. I'm sorry I'm a bit late for my appointment. The traffic outside is chaotic.

Dr. Bian: No problem. You're only a little late, and the traffic's always busy when the weather's bad. Anyway, we're planning to start the root canal treatment for your upper left molar today. How's the tooth been?

Mr. Wright: The tooth's been giving me some pain whenever I chew on that side. Otherwise, it's been okay. I'd like to know if it's really necessary to have the root canal treatment for this tooth. Can't you just put a filling in the cavity? I don't like the sound of this root canal treatment. It sounds painful.

Dr. Bian: I understand your concerns about the root canal treatment, Mr. Wright. However, the decay in that tooth is very extensive and has already reached the nerve. The tooth is now dead, and the infection inside it needs to be removed if you want to save the tooth. Otherwise, extracting the tooth is an option.

Mr. Wright: Okay, I want to keep my tooth, but how long will the root canal treatment take? Will I have pain after my appointment?

Dr. Bian: The root canal treatment will take a few appointments, each about an hour long. Sometimes, the tooth can be uncomfortable for 1 or 2 days after each appointment, but it's usually manageable with painkillers.

Mr. Wright: Why does it have to take so long? I'd prefer if everything could be finished in one visit.

Dr. Bian: I'd prefer to finish it in one visit too, but this tooth has 3 or 4 root canals. Each canal is quite small and curved, so it takes time to clean out each one thoroughly. While I'd like to be quick, it's important to be thorough to ensure the treatment is successful.

Mr. Wright: Thank you for explaining that. I'd rather have the treatment done right the first time and avoid needing it redone later.

Dr. Bian: Absolutely. Before we begin, I'll numb the tooth with a local anesthetic injection. Then I'll place a rubber dam around the tooth to isolate it. You'll need to breathe through your nose while I'm working.

Mr. Wright: Please go ahead.

📑 Treatment—Extraction

Mrs. Young: Dr. Hua, thank you for fitting me in this morning as an emergency. I broke a tooth last night eating some peanuts. It's been really painful since, and I couldn't sleep even after taking some painkillers.

Dr. Hua: Don't mention it. I always try to see a patient who's in pain. Can you recall any problems with your teeth before you broke this one? Which tooth did you break?

Mrs. Young: As far as I can remember, I haven't noticed any problems with my teeth before last night. But I haven't had a dental checkup for over a year. The painful tooth is on the lower left side—you'll see it as soon as you look inside my mouth. It feels very sharp to my tongue as well.

Dr. Hua: Okay, let me take a look.

(*After dental examination*)

Dr. Hua: Mrs. Young, I can see the tooth in question. It's suffered a serious fracture, and more than half of it is missing. The nerve is now exposed, which is likely the main reason you're in so much pain.

Mrs. Young: Can the tooth be saved? I don't want to lose it if possible.

Dr. Hua: It's possible to save the tooth, but it will require extensive treatment to stop the pain, rebuild the tooth, and make it strong enough to use. The tooth will need root canal treatment, a post and core, and finally a crown to protect it.

Mrs. Young: That sounds like a lot of work. How long will it take, and how much will it cost?

Dr. Hua: You'll need to come back for a few appointments—probably 4 or 5. As for the cost, my nurse will work out an estimate for you in a moment, but it's likely to be around 7 or 8 thousand yuan.

Mrs. Young: 4 or 5 appointments won't be too much of a problem, but the cost is quite high. How long do you think the tooth will last? Is it worth saving, in your opinion? What are the alternatives?

Dr. Hua: It's difficult to say exactly how long the tooth will last. It partly depends on how you use the tooth once the treatment is complete. It's kind of like when your car gets repaired—the mechanic can't guarantee how long it will last. In my opinion, I'd recommend extracting the tooth because the fracture line extends below the gum. You can then consider replacing it if necessary. The options include a denture, a bridge, or an implant. However, you don't need to decide on a replacement right away.

Mrs. Young: I'll take your advice and have the tooth extracted. Regarding the replacement, I'll decide later. Can you extract the tooth for me this morning?

Dr. Hua: I believe we can fit in the extraction this session. It's a busy morning, so I'll give you a local anesthetic first, and then you'll need to sit in the waiting room for a short time while I see some of my scheduled patients. Is that okay?

Mrs. Young: I'd be grateful if you could extract the tooth today. I don't mind waiting as you suggested.

Dr. Hua: Thank you for your understanding. From the medical form, I see you're fit and healthy and not taking any medication. Have you had breakfast this morning?

Mrs. Young: No, I've been in so much pain that I've lost my appetite completely.

Dr. Hua: In that case, my nurse will give you a glucose drink to boost your blood sugar level before the local anesthetic injections. I don't want you to faint during the treatment.

(*After local anesthetic injections*)

Dr. Hua: Has the toothache stopped, Mrs. Young? Does the area feel numb?

Mrs. Young: Yes, the whole lower left side feels very numb. How long will this last?

Dr. Hua: It usually lasts for 2 to 3 hours. You'll feel some pressure on the tooth now, but you shouldn't feel any sharp pain. Let me know if you do.

(*After extraction*)

Dr. Hua: Mrs. Young, the tooth has been extracted in one piece. I'm now squeezing the socket, and I'll ask you to bite firmly on a gauze pad for a few minutes to stop the bleeding.

(*After checking the socket*)

Dr. Hua: I've just checked the socket, and the bleeding has stopped. You can leave now, but I'd like you to bite on another piece of gauze for another 15 minutes. My nurse will give you a leaflet on what to do after an extraction. She'll also provide you with some extra gauze pads and painkiller tablets. Just be careful over the next few hours while your lip and tongue are still numb—it's easy to bite them accidentally. I suggest you come back in a week's time so I can check that the socket is healing properly. It's also a good idea to have your other teeth checked as well.

Mrs. Young: Thank you, doctor. I'll make an appointment outside.

▣ Treatment—Minor Oral Surgery

Dr. Cai: Hello, Mr. Olsen. How are you today?

Mr. Olsen: Hello. Thanks to the medicine you prescribed, I'm feeling much better than last week. However, I'm a bit wary of what you're going to do to me today.

Dr. Cai: That's understandable. However, I'm sure you're aware of the possibility of your wisdom tooth flaring up again if it's not removed. You certainly don't want to experience all that pain and swelling again.

Mr. Olsen: You're right. I suppose I'll have to get it done sooner or later. Would you mind just running through what you're going to do today?

Dr. Cai: No trouble at all. Your lower right wisdom tooth is partially erupted and isn't positioned correctly. From the radiograph, you can see it's pushing against the back of the tooth in front. Previously, you had a pretty nasty infection around this tooth, likely because it's difficult to keep that area clean. To prevent further problems, the tooth will need to be extracted. Since you're fit and healthy, I'd recommend doing it under local anesthetic right here in the surgery.

Mr. Olsen: Okay, is it possible to have a general anesthetic? Some of my friends told me they had their wisdom teeth taken out under general anesthetic when they were put to sleep.

Dr. Cai: In my opinion, a general anesthetic is advisable if the tooth is very difficult to remove or if the patient needs to have all four wisdom teeth extracted. In those cases, it might be easier for everyone involved to perform the operation under general anesthetic. However, you only need one tooth removed, and it's not particularly difficult. I'd advise that a local anesthetic is more appropriate. Additionally, with a general anesthetic, you usually have to stay in the hospital at least the night before and the night after the operation.

Mr. Olsen: That'd be inconvenient since I'd have to take time off, and it's very busy at work right now. Would I feel anything during the operation under local anesthetic? What exactly do you have to do?

Dr. Cai: No, the area I'm going to operate on will be completely numbed. You won't feel pain, but you might feel some vibration and pressure. After making sure you're numb, I'll need to cut into the gum and lift it to expose the wisdom tooth. It's usually necessary to remove some bone around the tooth with a drill. Ideally, the tooth is removed in one piece, but sometimes it needs to be sectioned into two or three pieces and removed individually. After that, I'll place a few sutures in the gums to ensure quick and trouble-free healing.

Mr. Olsen: Alright. I hope you don't mind, but I have just one more question. Have you done this type of operation before?

Dr. Cai: Yes, I've performed many wisdom tooth extractions similar to yours. You'll be in good hands.

Mr. Olsen: Thanks. Please go ahead.

(*After the extraction*)

Dr. Cai: I hope you're okay, Mr. Olsen. The tooth has been extracted, and I've put a few sutures in the area. You need to sit here for a while and bite on this piece of gauze. I'll check that your bleeding has stopped before we let you go.

(*After haemostasis*)

Dr. Cai: The bleeding has stopped now, and I'll see you at your appointment next week to remove the sutures. Please be careful with your numb lower lip and tongue. My nurse will give you some painkillers, extra gauze pads, and an instruction leaflet. There's an emergency phone number on the leaflet, just in case.

Mr. Olsen: Thank you very much, doctor. I didn't feel a thing. I'll see you next week.

📇 Treatment—Crown and Bridge

Dr. Bing: Hello, Mrs. Baker. Nice to see you again.

Mrs. Baker: Hello, Dr. Bing. I hope you're going to give me back my smile.

Dr. Bing: I'll do my best. As we discussed during your consultation, we'll replace your missing upper central incisor with a bridge. Once we fit the permanent bridge, you can finally throw away the denture you've been wearing for the past year!

Mrs. Baker: Yes, it'd be nice to get rid of the denture. It's starting to get a bit loose, and I haven't really enjoyed eating since I started wearing it. Would you mind just running through what you're going to do at this appointment?

Dr. Bing: Certainly. I'm going to prepare the two adjacent teeth to fit crowns over them. The bridge, as shown on this model, will have a porcelain tooth replacing the missing one, fused to the two crowns. The whole structure, comprising three units—two crowns and one replacement tooth—will be cemented onto the adjacent supporting teeth with permanent cement. Once it's in place, it'll feel like your own teeth.

Mrs. Baker: Will the bridge be ready today?

Dr. Bing: Unfortunately no. Each bridge is custom-made to fit the patient's mouth. After preparing the two supporting teeth today, I'll take some impressions of the teeth and gums. These impressions will be sent to the lab, where the technician will create plaster models and then make the bridge for you in the shade we chose at your last appointment. All these steps take time, and the finished product should be ready in about two weeks.

Mrs. Baker: Does that mean I'll have to keep my mouth closed all the time? I can't possibly see my friends with my teeth looking like small pegs.

Dr. Bing: Rest assured, Mrs. Baker, you'll still look presentable. I'll fit two temporary crowns over the adjacent teeth, but you'll have to keep using the denture for another two weeks until the bridge is ready. The temporary crowns will be cemented with a temporary cement, so you'll need to be careful with what you eat. They could get dislodged, although I can recement them if necessary. However, it might be inconvenient for you if they come loose unexpectedly. Also, please note that the temporary crowns might not be the exact color you want, as the choice of color is limited.

Mrs. Baker: Okay. Just one question before we start. Will I be in pain during or after the procedure?

Dr. Bing: The teeth will be numbed with a local anesthetic injection, so you shouldn't feel any pain during the procedure. However, they might be slightly sensitive to hot and cold for the next day or two. Most patients tolerate the sensitivity well, but painkillers like paracetamol or ibuprofen can help if needed. The chances of any serious pain are slim, but there's an emergency number printed on your appointment card. You can call it for advice or help if necessary. Do you have any other questions before we start?

Mrs. Baker: No, I'm fine now. Please go ahead, doctor.

Treatment—Denture

Dr. Wu: Good morning, Mr. Pang.

Mr. Pang: Hello, Dr. Wu. I'm having some problems with my dentures. The upper one has been repaired quite a few times, and they're starting to feel loose and uncomfortable to eat with.

Dr. Wu: How old is this set of dentures? If they were made a long time ago, they might not fit your mouth properly now. Over the years, your mouth changes shape, and the dentures can become uncomfortable.

Mr. Pang: I can't remember exactly how old this set is, but I'd guess at least 10 years old. They were made when I was still living in Beijing.

Dr. Wu: Let me take a look at the dentures in your mouth.

(*After oral examination*)

Mr. Pang: What do you think, doctor? Do I need a new set?

Dr. Wu: From what I can see, your upper full denture is starting to crack down the middle again. You might have a heavy bite, and the acrylic material of the denture isn't strong enough. Neither the upper nor lower dentures are fitting your mouth well. I imagine they move around when you try to chew. If they move excessively, you might develop ulcers where the dentures rub against your gums. I do think a new set of dentures is advisable.

Mr. Pang: How long would it take to make me a new set?

Dr. Wu: It would require several appointments, so at least 3 to 4 weeks. There are quite a few stages involved before the dentures are finally processed and ready for fitting.

Mr. Pang: Can you do anything to make this set more comfortable to wear in the meantime? I don't think I can put up with them for another month. They're just going to get more uncomfortable.

Dr. Wu: I can reline the dentures for you. This will make them a bit more comfortable while the new set is being made. However, I'll need to use your dentures to take some impressions of your jaws and send them to my technician for the reline. You'll be without your dentures for approximately a week. Will that be okay?

Mr. Pang: I suppose if there's no other option, I'll have to manage without them for a few days. But can we do the reline after this weekend? I have to attend a wedding banquet, and it's unthinkable for me to go without my dentures.

Dr. Wu: As you wish. We can arrange an appointment for you to come back on Monday. One more thing—since your upper denture has been repaired a few times, I would recommend using a metal plate in the palate of the new upper denture. It should strengthen that part of the denture and reduce the risk of it fracturing again.

Mr. Pang: That sounds like a good idea. I'd like that. So, I'll schedule an appointment to see you on Monday. See you then.

(沈雅修订)

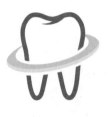

Part 2
Clinical
Presentations

Unit 2 ▶ The 'Normal' Dentitions

The first signs of tooth formation can be seen in the dental laminas when a foetus is 6-7 weeks old.

1. The Deciduous Dentition

At around 7 months of age the deciduous dentition begins to erupt, starting with the lower central and then the lateral incisors (Table 2.1). The teeth tend to be spaced and this spacing increase as the jaw grows. At 12-14 months of age the first deciduous molar (D) erupts, then the canines (C) at 18-20 months. The last tooth to erupt in the deciduous dentition is the second molar (E), which erupts between the ages of 2 and 3 years. The spacing is greatest in the maxilla distal to the lateral incisors. In the mandible the space is greatest distal to the canines. These widened gaps are known as the primate spaces [1]. The deciduous dentition often occludes edge-to-edge or nearly so and as toothwear occurs this tendency to an edge-to-edge occlusion increases.

Table 2.1   Development of the Primary Dentition

Tooth (in order of eruption)	Start of calcification	Eruption	Root completion (12-18 months after) eruption
Central incisors	14 weeks	6 months	2 years
Lateral incisors	14 weeks	7 months	2 years
First molars	15 weeks	12 months	2.5 years
Canines	16 weeks	18 months	3 years
Second molars	20 weeks	24 months (6-12 months' variation is normal)	4 years

(选自 *Dentistry at a Glance*, 1st Edition, Part 2, Chapter 26, Table 26.1)

本单元正文内容选自 Elizabeth Kay 所著 *Dentistry at a Glance*, John Wiley & Sons, Inc., 2016, Chapter 26, pp.56-57, 选用时图表序号有改动。

2. Eruption of Permanent Teeth

The lower central incisors erupt at around the age of 6 years and this coincides fairly closely with the eruption of all four first permanent molars (Table 2.2). This is followed by the eruption of the upper central and lower lateral incisors around the age of 7 years. The upper lateral incisors then appear at the age of 8 years (or thereabouts). The exact timing may vary somewhat, but the sequence of eruption is relatively ubiquitous. If the central incisor does not erupt in sequence, radiographs should be taken to ascertain whether a supernumerary or altered morphology is causing the delay [2].

The lower canine erupts between 9 and 10 years, as do the first premolar teeth. The upper canine and second premolars erupt at 11 and the second molars at 12. Both the presence and the eruption of third molars is very variable.

The deciduous molars are larger mesiodistally than the permanent premolars which replace them [3]. This is known as the 'leeway space' (width of C + D + E-width of 3 + 4 + 5) and is usually 1.5 mm in the upper and 2.5 mm in the lower [4].

Table 2.2　Development of the Secondary Dentition

Tooth (in order of eruption)	Start of calcification (5-6 years prior to eruption)	Eruption (+1)	Root completion (3+ years after eurption)
First molar	Birth	6 years	9 years
Mandibular central incisors	3 months	7 years	10 years
Maxillary central and mandibular lateral incisors	3 months	8 years	11 years
Maxillary lateral incisors	12 months	9 years	12 years
Mandibular canines	4 months	10 years	13 years
Maxillary first premolars	18 months	11 years	14 years
Mandibular first premolars	22 months	11 years	14 years
Maxillary canines	4 months	12 years	15 years
Maxillary second premolars	24 months	11 years	14 years
Mandibular second premolars	28 months	12 years	15 years
Second molars	32 months	12 years	15 years
Third molars	Variable	Variable	Variable

(选自 *Dentistry at a Glance*, 1st Edition, Part 2, Chapter 26, Table 26.2)

2.1　Stages of Eruption

There are four stages to the eruption of the permanent teeth.

Stage 1: As soon as root development begins, eruption starts. At the same time, resorption of the bone (and in the case of secondary teeth the primary tooth roots) needs to occur. If the two processes do not coincide, eruption will not progress.

Stage 2: When the root is about two-thirds complete, the tooth erupts into the mouth. The tooth moves approximately 0.4 mm/week and continues to erupt until aligned with the occlusal plane.

Stage 3: The maxilla and mandible continue to grow after the teeth have erupted into position and teeth continue to erupt to keep pace with this, with a speeding up of the eruption rate at the time of the adolescent growth spurt.

Stage 4: Teeth continue to erupt to compensate for occlusal wear and further growth. If there are no opposing teeth, over eruption will occur.

2.2 Early Mixed Dentition

The mixed dentition phase commences when the first permanent teeth, the mandibular lower incisors, erupt. The incisors often erupt slightly lingually to the deciduous tooth. As the upper centrals erupt, because of the position of the canine tooth close to the root of the lateral incisor, the lateral incisors are often distally inclined [5]. This is a normal stage of development, commonly (and rather unfairly!) called the 'ugly duckling stage' (Figure 2.1).

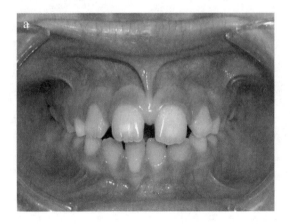 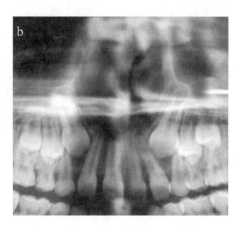

Figure 2.1 The ugly duckling stage of dental development: (a) the maxillary lateral incisors are distally splayed and there is a midline diastema; (b) the radiograph shows that the distal splaying is due to pressure on the lateral incisor roots by the developing canines.

Source: Gill D. (2008) *Orthodontics at a Glance*. Reproduced with permission of John Wiley & Sons, Inc.

（选自 *Dentistry at a Glance*, 1st Edition, Part 2, Chapter 26, Figure 26.1）

The permanent incisors are considerably bigger that the deciduous ones. They are accommodated partly because of the spacing found between deciduous incisors and by being slightly more proclined than the very upright deciduous teeth. There is also an increase in intercanine width—in the mandible due to the permanent canine erupting to occupy the primate space. There is, therefore, often some incisor crowding until the canines erupt.

2.3 Late Mixed Dentition

This phase begins when the lower canine erupts, along with the premolar teeth, around the age of 11 years. The upper canines should be palpable buccally from the age of about 9 years. Because they erupt after the upper premolars, any shortage of space will cause them to be crowded out of the arch [6]. If the canines erupt successfully, the incisors become less splayed and small diastemas will be likely to close.

📄 **Word List**

1. lamina [ˈlæmɪnə] *n.* 叶片;薄层;薄板
2. foetus [ˈfiːtəs] *n.* 胎儿
3. deciduous dentition 乳牙列
4. maxilla [mækˈsɪlə] *n.* 上颌骨
5. mandible [ˈmændɪbl] *n.* 下颌骨
6. primate spaces 灵长类间隙
7. ubiquitous [juːˈbɪkwɪtəs] *adj.* 无处不在的;普遍存在的
8. supernumerary [ˌsuːpəˈnjuːmərərɪ] *n.* 多生牙 *adj.* 多余的;过剩的
9. morphology [mɔːˈfɒlədʒɪ] *n.* 形态学
10. canine [ˈkeɪnaɪn] *n.* 尖牙
11. mesiodistally [ˌmɛsɪə(ʊ)ˈdɪstəlɪ] *adv.* 近远中方向地
12. leeway space 替牙间隙
13. occlusal plane 咬合平面
14. adolescent [ˌædəˈlesnt] *n.* 青少年
15. occlusal wear 咬合磨损
16. opposing teeth 对颌牙
17. mixed dentition 混合牙列
18. commence [kəˈmens] *vt.* 开始
19. ugly duckling stage 丑小鸭时期

📝 Notes

① These widened gaps are known as the primate spaces.

上颌乳尖牙近中面和下颌乳尖牙远中面的间隙称为灵长类间隙。

② If the central incisor does not erupt in sequence, radiographs should be taken to ascertain whether a supernumerary or altered morphology is causing the delay.

如果中切牙没有按顺序萌出，则应拍 X 线片以确定是否有多生牙或形态改变导致了迟萌。

③ The deciduous molars are larger mesiodistally than the permanent premolars which replace them.

乳磨牙比替换后的恒前磨牙在近远中方向上更大。

④ This is known as the 'leeway space' (width of C + D + E-width of 3 + 4 + 5) and is usually 1.5 mm in the upper and 2.5 mm in the lower.

这个宽度称为"替牙间隙"，即：替牙间隙 = (C+D+E) - (3+4+5)。在上颌约有 1.5mm，在下颌为 2mm。

⑤ As the upper centrals erupt, because of the position of the canine tooth close to the root of the lateral incisor, the lateral incisors are often distally inclined.

由于尖牙的位置靠近侧切牙的根部，所以上颌中切牙萌出时，侧切牙牙冠往往向远端倾斜。

⑥ Because they erupt after the upper premolars, any shortage of space will cause them to be crowded out of the arch.

由于上颌尖牙的萌出晚于上颌前磨牙，任何空间的不足都会导致它们被挤出牙弓。

（本单元由边专、贾荣选编）

（文字部分选自 *Dentistry at a Glance*，1st Edition，Part 2，Chapter 26）

Unit 3 ▶ Tooth Eruption and Exfoliation

1. Tooth Eruption

The process of eruption involves the movement or change of position of the tooth from the deeper portion of the jaws into the oral cavity until it achieves occlusal contact with adjacent and opposing teeth. Tooth eruption has three broad stages. The first, known as **primary dentition** stage, occurs when only primary teeth are visible. Once the first permanent tooth erupts into the mouth, the teeth are in the **mixed** (or transitional) **dentition**. After the last primary tooth falls out of the mouth, the teeth are in the **permanent dentition**. The chronological course of development for primary and permanent teeth is shown in Tables 3.1 and 3.2.

Table 3.1 The Chronological Course of Deciduous Tooth Development

Tooth type	Calcification begins		Crown completed		Eruption		Root completed	
	Maxillary (months in utero)	Mandibular (months in utero)	Maxillary (age in months)	Mandibular (age in months)	Maxillary (age in months)	Mandibular (age in months)	Maxillary (age in years)	Mandibular (age in years)
Central	3.5	3.5	1.5	2.5	10	7	1.5	1.5
Lateral	4	4	2.5	3	11	13	2	1.5
Canine	4.25	4.25	9	9	19	20	3.25	3.25
1st Molar	3.75	3.75	6	5.5	16	16	2.5	2.25
2nd Molar	4.75	4.5	12	10	29	27	3	3

(选自 *Dentistry at a Glance*, 1st Edition, Part 2, Chapter 31, Table 31.1)

本单元正文内容选自 Elizabeth Kay 所著 *Dentistry at a Glance*, John Wiley & Sons, Inc., 2016, Chapter 31, pp.68-69。

Table 3.2　The Chronological Course of Deciduous Tooth Development

Tooth type	Calcification begins		Crown completed		Eruption		Root completed	
	Maxillary	Mandibular	Maxillary (years)	Mandibular (years)	Maxillary (years)	Mandibular (years)	Maxillary (years)	Mandibular (years)
Central	3–4 months	3–4 months	4–5	3.5–4.5	6.5–8	5.5–7	10–11	9–10
Lateral	10–12 months	3–4 months	4.5–5.5	4–5	7.5–9	7–8	11	10
Canine	4–5 months	4–5 months	6–7	5.5–6.5	11–12	9–10	13–15	12–14
1st Premolar	18–22 months	18–22 months	5.5–7	5–6.75	9.5–11	10–12	12–14	12–14
2nd Premolar	24–27 months	24–27 months	6–7	6–7	10–12	10.5–12	12–14.5	13–15
1st molar	at birth	at birth	2.5–4	2.5–3.75	5.5–7	5–7	9–11	9–11
2nd molar	29 months	29 months	7–8	7–8	12–13	11–13	14–16	14–16
3rd molar	7–9 years	8–10 years	12–16	12–16	17–22	17–22	18–25	18–25

（选自 *Dentistry at a Glance*，1st Edition，Part 2，Chapter 31，Table 31.2）

1.1　Rate of Tooth Eruption

The rate of eruption represents a balance between forces tending to move the tooth into the mouth (**eruptive force**) and forces tending to prevent this movement (**resistive force**). Resistance may be produced by overlying soft tissues and alveolar bone, the viscosity of the surrounding periodontal ligament and occlusal forces. However, little is known about the nature, source and magnitude of either the eruptive or resistive forces [1].

The rate of tooth eruption also depends on the phase of movement. In the **intraosseous phase**, the rate of tooth eruption is 1-10 μm/day; in the **extraosseous phase** it is 75 μm/day. It takes approximately 2-3 years after eruption for permanent teeth to finish calcification. In radiographic studies it was found that the interval between crown completion and beginning of eruption until the tooth is in full occlusion is approximately 5-6 years for permanent teeth.

1.2　Mechanism of Tooth Movements

Tooth eruption is traditionally considered to be a developmental process. However, eruption can be regarded as a lifelong process because a tooth will often move axially in response to changing functional situations. This is shown in overeruption, resulting from the removal of an opposite tooth, or compensatory eruption related to attrition.

The theories advanced to explain the mechanism of tooth eruption can be divided into two main groups: (1) the tooth is pushed out as a result of forces generated beneath and around it, either by alveolar bone growth, root growth, blood-pressure/ tissue fluid pressure, or cell proliferation [2]; and (2) the tooth may be pulled out as a result of tension within the connective tissue of the periodontal ligament. Although the exact mechanism of eruption is still debatable, there are four important factors that are considered to be responsible for the eruption of teeth:

- Bone remodelling (deposition vs. resorption)
- Root growth
- Vascular (hydrostatic) pressure
- Periodontal ligament traction.

1.3　Sequence of Eruption

The eruption or appearance of the teeth follows a general pattern or schedule. In general, the mandibular teeth precede the maxillary teeth. Homologous teeth in the same arch erupt at roughly the same time. A time period of more than 6 months between the eruption of homologous teeth should not be considered normal [3].

- The most common eruption sequence of the primary dentition is:

$$\frac{AB \quad D \quad C \quad E}{A \quad B \quad D \quad CE}$$

- The most common eruption sequence of the permanent dentition is:

$$\frac{6 \quad 1 \quad 2 \quad 4 \quad 5 \quad 3 \quad 7 \quad 8}{6 \quad 1 \quad 2 \quad 3 \quad 4 \quad 5 \quad 7 \quad 8}$$

2.　Exfoliation of Primary Teeth

The physiological process responsible for the loss of deciduous or primary teeth is known as exfoliation or shedding. The roots of primary teeth begin to resorb approximately 3 years after completion. Resorption of a primary tooth root is the gradual dissolving away of the root due to the underlying eruption of the successors that will replace it. Root resorption continues as the successors move closer to the surface until the primary teeth eventually become loose and finally fall out [4]. When a primary tooth is shed, the crown of the successors is close to the surface and ready to emerge. The interval between shedding of the primary teeth and emergence of the permanent teeth is usually 3-6 months [5].

2.1　Pattern of Resorption and Shedding

For a primary incisor or canine, root resorption initially occurs on the lingual surface adjacent to the developing permanent tooth. With subsequent movement and relocation of the teeth in the growing jaws, the developing permanent tooth comes to lie directly beneath the primary tooth and further resorption occurs from the apex. For a primary molar, root resorption often commences on the inner surfaces where the permanent premolars initially develop. The premolars later come to lie beneath the roots of the primary molar and further resorption occurs from the root apices. The shift in position of the primary tooth relative to the permanent successor may account for the intermittent nature of root resorption.

2.2　Mechanism of Resorption and Shedding

The initiation of root resorption may be an inherent developmental process, or it may be related to pressure from the permanent successor against the overlying bone or tooth. To examine which of these theories is correct, researchers have surgically removed permanent tooth germs and found that resorption of the predecessors still occurred, though the resortion process was delayed. This finding is also consistent with the clinical observation that shedding of a primary tooth still occurs but is retarded where the successor is congenitally missing (Figure 3.1), impacted or ectopically positioned. In this case, a primary tooth may exfoliate when the patient is older than 30 years.

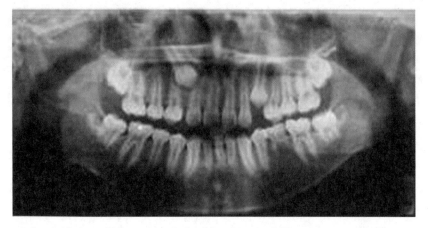

Figure 3.1　A 12-year-old boy with missing 35 and retained 75; other premolars have erupted.
(选自 *Dentistry at a Glance*, 1st Edition, Part 2, Chapter 36, Figure 31.1)

It has also been suggested that increased masticatory loads may affect the pattern and rate of primary tooth resorption [6]. It has been shown in experiment that, if primary teeth were splinted following the removal of the developing permanent teeth, there was less root resorption compared with removal of the permanent teeth alone.

📄 Word List

1. exfoliation [ˌeksˌfəʊlɪˈeɪʃn] *n.* 脱落
2. occlusal contact 咬合接触
3. primary dentition 乳牙列
4. permanent dentition 恒牙列
5. chronological [ˌkrɒnəˈlɒdʒɪkl] *adj.* 按时间先后的
6. viscosity [vɪˈskɒsətɪ] *n.* 黏性；黏度；黏滞物
7. periodontal ligament 牙周膜；牙周膜韧带
8. occlusal forces 咬合力
9. attrition [əˈtrɪʃn] *n.* 磨损
10. deposition [ˌdepəˈzɪʃn] *n.* 沉积
11. hydrostatic [ˌhaɪdrəˈstætɪk] *adj.* 流体静力的
12. homologous [həˈmɒləɡəs] *adj.* 同源的；类似的
13. lingual [ˈlɪŋɡwəl] *adj.* 舌侧的
14. congenitally [kənˈdʒenɪtəlɪ] *adv.* 天生地；先天地

📝 Notes

❶ However, little is known about the nature, source and magnitude of either the eruptive or resistive forces.
然而，人们对促进牙齿萌出的力或阻力的性质、来源和强度知之甚少。

❷ the tooth is pushed out as a result of forces generated beneath and around it, either by alveolar bone growth, root growth, blood-pressure/ tissue fluid pressure, or cell proliferation.
牙齿萌出来自其下方和周围的力量：牙槽骨生长、牙根生长、血压/组织液压力或细胞增殖等作用。

❸ A time period of more than 6 months between the eruption of homologous teeth should not be considered normal.

同颌同名牙萌出时间间隔超过 6 个月被认为是不正常的。

❹ Root resorption continues as the successors move closer to the surface until the primary teeth eventually become loose and finally fall out.

随着继承恒牙逐渐萌出接近咬合平面, 乳牙牙根开始吸收并最终松动脱落。

❺ The interval between shedding of the primary teeth and emergence of the permanent teeth is usually 3-6 months.

牙脱落和恒牙萌出的间隔一般是 3~6 个月。

❻ It has also been suggested that increased masticatory loads may affect the pattern and rate of primary tooth resorption.

也有人认为咀嚼负荷的增加可能会影响乳牙吸收的模式和速度。

（本单元由贾荣选编）

（文字部分选自 *Dentistry at a Glance*, 1st Edition, Part 2, Chapter 31）

Unit 4 ▶ Properties of Tooth Tissue

A thorough understanding of the anatomy and biology of the tooth is necessary for successful clinical dentistry. Dentistry that violates the physical, chemical and biological parameters of the tooth tissue can lead to premature restoration failure, compromised coronal integrity, recurrent caries, patient discomfort or pulpal necrosis [1].

1. Enamel

Enamel provides a hard durable surface to protect the dentine and pulp. Its form and colour also has a major role in aesthetics (Figure 4.1); therefore, the lifelong preservation of the patient's own enamel is one of the goals of modern dentistry.

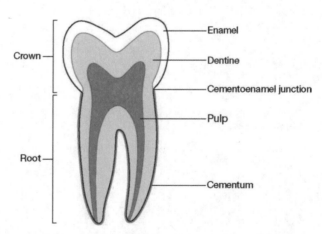

Figure 4.1　Schematic view of the tooth structure

（选自 *Dentistry at a Glance*, 1st Edition, Part 2, Chapter 38, Figure 38.1）

本单元正文内容选自 Elizabeth Kay 所著 *Dentistry at a Glance*, John Wiley & Sons, Inc., 2016, Chapter 38, pp.84-85, 选用时图表序号有改动。

1.1 Permeability

The water in enamel (Table 4.1) is contained within the intercrystalline spaces and in a network of micropores opening to the external surface, which makes enamel a semipermeable material.

Table 4.1 Enamel Properties

Compostition(by volume)	
Inorganic hydroxyapatie	86%
Water	4%-12%
Organic matrix	Trace
Thickness(mm)	
Cusp tips	2.5
Incisal edge	2.0
Cervical areas	minimal to nil
Occlusal fissures	minimal to nil

(选自 *Dentistry at a Glance*, 1st Edition, Part 2, Chapter 38, Box 38.1)

1.2 Colour

Enamel translucency is directly related to its degree of mineralisation and thickness. The colour of the tooth is determined by the colour of the underlying dentine as well as the translucency of the enamel covering it.

1.3 Wear

Enamel is a hard material but it wears when it is opposed by enamel or harder restorative materials (e.g., porcelain) [2].

1.4 Acid Etching

Enamel is differentially soluble when exposed for a brief time to weak acids. This process is called acid etching and approximately 10 μm of surface enamel (but no rod structures) is removed. If acid exposure continues, the differential dissolution of enamel rod and inter-rod structures forms a three-dimensional macroporous structure, which can be used to attract resin monomer during restorative bonding procedures.

2. Dentine

The coronal dentine is covered by enamel and forms the bulk of the structure of the tooth. This dentine is responsible for protecting the pulp as well as forming an elastic foundation to support the enamel and dictate the overall tooth shade. The radicular dentine is covered by cementum and forms the roots. Dentine is capable of responding to external thermal, chemical and mechanical stimuli.

2.1 Support

The strength, rigidity and integrity of the tooth rely on an intact dentinal structure. When a tooth is prepared for restoration, its resistance to fracture decreases. Removal and replacement of dental restorations result in progressively larger or deeper restorations throughout the patient's life.

2.2 Morphology

Dentine is composed of small, thin apatite crystal flakes embedded in a protein matrix of cross-linked collagen fibrils (Table 4.2). Two main types of dentine are present: intertubular dentine, which forms the bulk of the dentine structure and is composed of a hydroxyapatite-embedded collagen matrix, and peritubular dentine, which is limited to the lining of the dentinal tubule walls. It has little organic matrix and is packed with miniscule apatite crystals.

Table 4.2 Dentine Properties

Composition(by volume)	
Inorganic apatite crystals	45%–50%
Organic matrix	30%
Water	25%
Rate of secretion(μm/day)	
Primary dentine	4–8
Secondary dentine	1–2

（选自 *Dentistry at a Glance*，1st Edition Part 2，Chapter 38，Box 38.2）

2.3 Permeability

The dentinal tubules have a functional role in forming and maintaining the dentine but, when exposed, they make the dentine permeable (Figure 4.2).

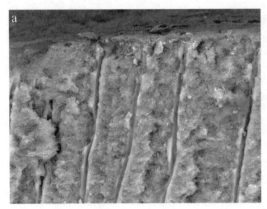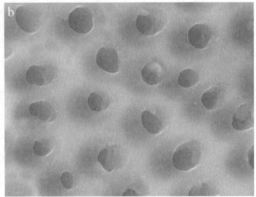

Figure 4.2 （a）Cross section of the dentinal tubules；（b）when the smear layer is removed, the dentinal tubules can act as passages between the oral environment and the pulp.

Source：Reproduced with permission from Dr. Nikolas Silikas.

（选自 *Dentistry at a Glance*，1st Edition，Part 2，Chapter 38，Figure 38.2）

2.4 Primary and Secondary Dentine

Once the odontoblast cells are differentiated from ectomesenchymal cells, they start secreting an organic matrix. This matrix mineralises and forms the primary dentine. Approximately 2 to 3 years following tooth eruption, the synthesis of the dentine slows down and continues for as long as the tooth is vital. This dentine is called secondary dentine and is responsible for reducing the size of the pulp chamber [3].

2.5 Tertiary Dentine

When dentine is lost due to caries or injury, new dentine (tertiary dentine) will form at the dentine-pulp interface if the tooth retains its vitality. If the stimulus is low grade, this dentine is made by the odontoblasts and is called reactionary dentine. If the stimulus is severe or the thickness of the remaining dentine falls below 0.25 mm, the odontoblasts will die. The stem cells within the vital pulp will form odontoblast-like cells, which will then create a bridge of dentine. This dentine is called reparative dentine.

3. Pulp

Dental pulp is composed of 75% water and 25% organic material, which form a viscous connective tissue of collagen fibres and organic ground substance which supports the cellular, vascular and nerve structures of the tooth.

The dental pulp has several functions:

3.1 Formative

Odontolasts within the dental pulp are responsible for generating primary, secondary and tertiary dentine. They also produce growth factors and bioactive signalling molecules, which coordinates the pulpal-dentinal responses for healing and repair. Fibroblasts produce, maintain and remodel pulp matrix and collagen.

3.2 Nutritive

The microvascular system of the pulp contains vessels no larger than arterioles and venules. Lymphatic vessels of the pulp return tissue fluid and high molecular-weight plasma proteins back to the vascular system [4]. The transfer of the oxygen, nutrition and waste materials is done by diffusion within the viscous ground substance of the pulp.

3.3 Sensory

The majority of the nerve fibres are either A-δ or unmyelinated C fibres. The A-δ nerves react to hydrodynamic phenomena and their activation results in sharp and intense pain. The C fibres, however, are only activated by a level of stimuli that is capable of creating tissue destruction (i.e., prolonged high temperature or pulpitis). The pain is diffuse in nature and described as burning or throbbing, which may be difficult to locate. The C fibres are resistant to hypoxia and are not affected by reduction of blood flow or high tissue pressure; therefore, pain may persist in anaesthetised, infected or even non-vital teeth [5].

3.4 Protective

The immunocompetent cells within the pulp consist of macrophages, lymphocytes and dendritic cells. These cells function as a host defense system against foreign bodies and antigens.

4. Cementum

Cementum is the calcified, avascular mesenchymal tissue that forms the outer covering of the anatomic root. The two main types of cementum are acellular (primary) and cellular (secondary) and both consist of a calcified interfibrillar matrix and collagen fibrils. The two main sources of collagen fibres in cementum are Sharpey's fibres (extrinsic), which are the embedded portion of the principal fibres of the periodontal ligament and are formed by fibroblasts, and fibres that belong to the cementum matrix (intrinsic) and are produced by the cementoblasts [6].

4.1 Permeability

Cementum is very permeable in young teeth but this diminishes with age.

4.2　Cementoenamel Junction (CEJ)

Three types of CEJ may exist (Table 4.3). When there is a gap between enamel and cementum, gingival recession may result in exposed dentine and sensitivity.

Table 4.3　Types of CEJ

Cementum-enamel relationships	
Cementum overlaps enamel	60%-65%
Edge-to-edge	30%
Cementum does not meet enamel	5%-10%

(选自 *Dentistry at a Glance*,1st Edition, Part 2, Chapter 38, Box 38.3)

4.3　Cementum Resorption

Primary teeth undergo physiological resorption; however, in adult teeth cementum resorption may occur due to local or systemic factors (Table 4.4) or may occur without apparent aetiology (idiopathic). In rare cases of resorption, cementum and root can be gradually replaced by bone, resulting in ankylosis. An ankylosed tooth lacks physiological mobility and makes a metallic sound on percussion [7].

Table 4.4　Factors Causing Resorption of Cementum

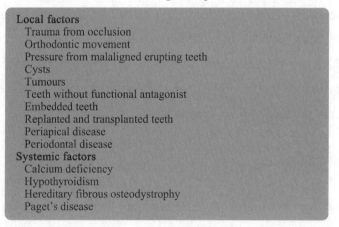

Local factors
 Trauma from occlusion
 Orthodontic movement
 Pressure from malaligned erupting teeth
 Cysts
 Tumours
 Teeth without functional antagonist
 Embedded teeth
 Replanted and transplanted teeth
 Periapical disease
 Periodontal disease
Systemic factors
 Calcium deficiency
 Hypothyroidism
 Hereditary fibrous osteodystrophy
 Paget's disease

(选自 *Dentistry at a Glance*,1st Edition, Part 2, Chapter 38, Box 38.4)

📄 Word List

1. enamel [ɪˈnæml] *n.* 搪瓷；珐琅；瓷釉；釉质；指甲油
2. semipermeable [ˈsemɪˈpɜːmɪəbl] *adj.* 半渗透的
3. etching [ˈetʃɪŋ] *n.* 蚀刻术；蚀刻版画
4. microporous [ˈmaɪkrəʊˈpɔːrəs] *adj.* 大孔的；大孔隙的；多孔的
5. dentine [ˈdentiːn] *n.* 牙质；牙本质
6. radicular [ræˈdɪkjʊlə(r)] *adj.* 根的；小根的
7. intertubular [ɪntɜːˈtjuːbjʊlə] *adj.* 管间的
8. hydroxyapatite [ˌhaɪdrɒksɪˈæpətaɪt] *n.* [矿物]羟基磷灰石
9. tertiary [ˈtɜːʃərɪ] *adj.* 第三的；第三位的；第三级的
10. aetiology [ˌiːtiˈɒlədʒɪ] *n.* [基医]病因学；病原学；原因论
11. ankylosis [ˌæŋkɪˈləʊsɪs] *n.* [外科]关节僵硬；胶着

✏️ Notes

❶ Dentistry that violates the physical, chemical and biological parameters of the tooth tissue can lead to premature restoration failure, compromised coronal integrity, recurrent caries, patient discomfort or pulpal necrosis.
违背牙组织的物理、化学和生物参数的牙科治疗，可导致牙体修复过早失败、牙冠完整性受损、继发龋、患者不适或牙髓坏死。

❷ Enamel is a hard material but it wears when it is opposed by enamel or harder restorative materials (e.g. porcelain).
牙釉质是一种坚硬的材料，但当它与牙釉质或更硬的修复材料(比如瓷)咬合时，它会磨损。

❸ Once the odontoblast cells are differentiated from ectomesenchymal cells, they start secreting an organic matrix. This matrix mineralises and forms the primary dentine. Approximately 2 to 3 years following tooth eruption, the synthesis of the dentine slows down and continues for as long as the tooth is vital. This dentine is called secondary dentine and is responsible for reducing the size of the pulp chamber.

一旦成牙本质细胞从外胚间充质细胞分化出来，它们就开始分泌有机基质。这种基质矿化并形成原发性牙本质。牙齿长出后 2 到 3 年，牙本质的合成会减慢，只要牙齿还能发挥作用，这种现象就会持续下去，这类牙本质被称为继发性牙本质，会牵连减小牙髓腔的体积。

❹　The microvascular system of the pulp contains vessels no larger than arterioles and venules. Lymphatic vessels of the pulp return tissue fluid and high molecular-weight plasma proteins back to the vascular system.

牙髓的微血管系统包含比小动脉和小静脉还小的血管。牙髓的淋巴管将组织液和高分子量血浆蛋白送回血管系统。

❺　The C fibres are resistant to hypoxia and are not affected by reduction of blood flow or high tissue pressure; therefore, pain may persist in anaesthetised, infected or even non-vital teeth.

C 纤维对缺氧具有抵抗力，不受血流减少或高组织压力的影响；因此，麻醉、感染甚至无活力的牙仍可能持续疼痛。

❻　The two main sources of collagen fibres in cementum are Sharpey's fibres (extrinsic), which are the embedded portion of the principal fibres of the periodontal ligament and are formed by fibroblasts, and fibres that belong to the cementum matrix (intrinsic) and are produced by the cementoblasts.

牙骨质中的胶原纤维主要有两种来源：一种是 Sharpey 纤维（外源性的），它是牙周膜主要纤维的嵌入部分，由成纤维细胞形成；另一种是属于牙骨质基质的纤维（内源性的），由成牙骨质细胞产生。

❼　In rare cases of resorption, cementum and root can be gradually replaced by bone, resulting in ankylosis. An ankylosed tooth lacks physiological mobility and makes a metallic sound on percussion.

在少数牙骨质吸收情况下，牙骨质及牙根会逐渐被骨质取代，形成牙齿固连。发生固连的牙会失去生理动度，敲击时有金属声。

（本单元由季耀庭选编）

（文字部分选自 *Dentistry at a Glance*，1st Edition, Part 2, Chapter 38）

Unit 5 ▶ Caries

Dental caries develops where biofilms form from deposits of microbes (Figure 5.1). This occurs at sites in the dentition where mechanical action fails to remove bacteria.

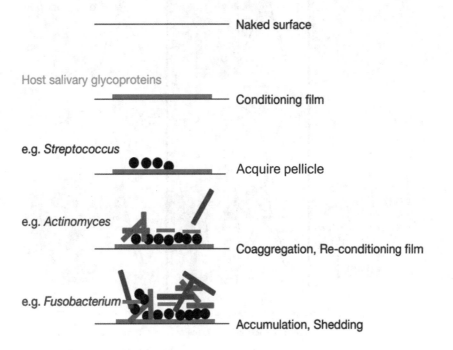

Figure 5.1   Stages in the formation of an oral biofilm community.

Source: Lamont R. J. (2010). *Oral Microbiology at a Glance*. Reproduced with permission of John Wiley & Sons, Inc.

(选自 *Dentistry at a Glance*, 1st Edition, Part 2, Chapter 32, Figure 32.1)

本单元正文内容选自 Elizabeth Kay 所著 *Dentistry at a Glance*, John Wiley & Sons, Inc., 2016, Chapter 32, pp.70-72, 选用时图表序号有改动。

1.　What Happens?

After a week of enamel being in juxtaposition with an undisturbed biofilm, although no changes would be seen clinically, microscopically the outer enamel surface can be seen to have signs of dissolution, making the enamel slightly more porous [1] (Figure 5.2).

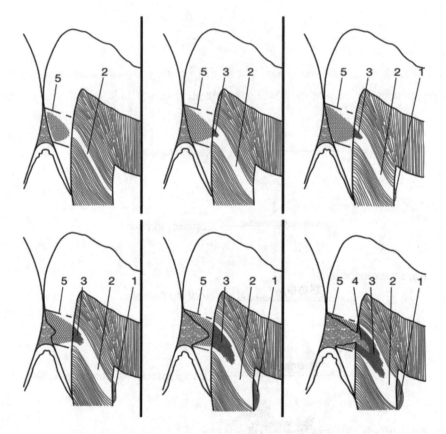

Figure 5.2　Schematic illustration of progressive stages of lesion formation

(1) Reactive dentine; (2) sclerotic reaction or translucent (transparent) zone; (3) zone of demineralisation; (4) zone of bacterial invasion and destruction; (5) peripheral rod direction.

Source: Fejerskov O. et al. (2008) In: Fejerskov O., Kidd E. (eds.) *Dental Caries: The Disease and Its Clinical Management* (2nd edn.). Reproduced with permission of John Wiley and Sons, Inc.

（选自 *Dentistry at a Glance*, 1st Edition Part 2, Chapter 32, Figure 32.2）

After 14 days, with completely undisturbed plaque, the enamel will appear whitish and opaque to the naked eye after air drying. This is because the enamel porosity has increased some more, but this time the porosity has increased because mineral underneath the outer surface has been preferentially removed, creating a subsurface lesion.

After 4 weeks, an active enamel lesion, or white-spot lesion, will have a chalky surface because the demineralisation and increased porosity cause loss of translucency [3]. It is also partly due to surface erosion. At this stage, careful brushing to remove plaque can reverse the process and surface hardness can be recovered.

2. Dentine Reactions to Enamel Lesions

The dentine underneath the enamel lesion will be the first to show signs of tubular sclerosis. When the enamel lesion reaches the enamel-dentine junction, demineralisation of the dentine along the junction occurs.

3. Lesion Progression

Whilst subsurface mineral loss occurs, the enamel is still a highly mineralized tissue, which is called undermining caries. Surface breakdown appears to occur due to the demineralized enamel being traumatized. This is why it is particularly important not to disturb enamel surfaces with a probe as this will introduce bacteria into the microcavity created by the probe tip, thereby transforming a demineralized area into a cavity. Once the microcavity is formed, bacteria will lodge within it and will be unlikely to be dislodged by mechanical cleaning.

Thus, the enamel cavity is enlarged by the combined effect of acid production by undisturbed bacteria and mechanical breakdown.

Following exposure of the dentine to the bacteria in the cavity (which is still confined to enamel), the most superficial dentine is relatively easily damaged by the acids being produced. After this, the bacteria invade the dentinal tubules (Figure 5.3).

4. Pulp Reaction

The pulp can stimulate reactionary or reparative dentine to form even before the bacterial invasion reaches the dentine. When the demineralisation of the dentine reaches 0.5-1 mm from the pulp, an inflammatory reaction in the pulp will occur. The pulp is not yet infected but the pulp reacts to bacterial products.

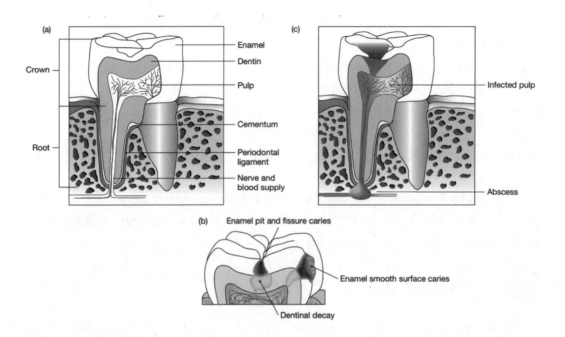

Figure 5.3

(a) Vertical sections showing major components of the tooth; (b) caries begins as reversible demineralisation (white spot); (c) if demineralisation continues the enamel decays and destruction eventually spreads through the dentine to the pulp chamber, which can lead to a periapical abscess

Source: Lamont R. J. (2010). *Oral Microbiology at a Glance*. Reproduced with permission of John Wiley & Sons, Inc.

(选自 *Dentistry at a Glance*, 1st Edition, Part 2, Chapter 32, Figure 32.3)

5. Microbiology of Caries

More than 700 different types of bacteria have been detected in the mouth. Different areas of the mouth are populated by different types of bacteria. The mouth is largely an aerobic environment but anaerobic bacteria can exist in biofilms on oral surfaces. The bacteria have to bond to a surface in order not to be washed away with saliva and ultimately ingested.

Carbohydrates increase the growth of many oral bacteria and increase acid production. This in turn makes the environment conducive to the more acidophilic bacteria.

5.1 Biofilm Formation in the Mouth

Teeth are covered by a film known as the acquired pellicle. This film is comprised of glycoproteins, phosphoproteins, lipids and other materials and may be 1μm thick after a period of 24 hours. It appears that bacteria are initially attracted to the tooth's pellicle by weak physicochemical forces but then adhesins on the cell wall interact with the pellicle.

The first colonisers of the tooth surface are usually *Streptococcus. sanguinis*, *S. oralis*, and *S. mitis* alongside *Actinomyces* and Gram-negative bacteria such as *Haemophilus*.

As the biofilm ages, the biomass ceases to be largely *streptococci* and becomes dominated by *Actinomyces*—a process known as microbial succession. As the bacterial deposits increase, the oxygen concentration lessens—thus plaque on teeth starts life composed of aerobic species but increasingly shifts to being made up of greater numbers of facultative anaerobes [2].

5.2 Bacteria and Non-milk Extrinsic Sugars

Some acid-producing bacteria are found in dental biofilms, but if the pH is neutral, they form only a small proportion of the total biomass. Whilst this is the case, any acid produced as a result of bacterial activity is minimal and its demineralisation effect can be counteracted. Thus demineralisation and remineralisation are in equilibrium. However, when non-milk extrinsic sugars (NMES) are eaten, or if salivary flow reduces, pH may fall below pH 5.5 (the critical point for demineralisation) for a sufficient amount of time for enamel demineralisation to occur. This has two effects. The low pH encourages the growth of acid-loving and producing bacteria (*mutans streptococci* and *lactobacilli*) and continues to favour demineralisation. *Mutans streptococci* and *lactobacilli*, in turn, cause more acid to be produced at a greater rate and thus demineralisation is further favoured. Thus, caries is a result of a change in the balance of the bacterial ecology, which comes about because the oral environment has changed (that is, become more acid because excess NMES is available) (Figure 5.4).

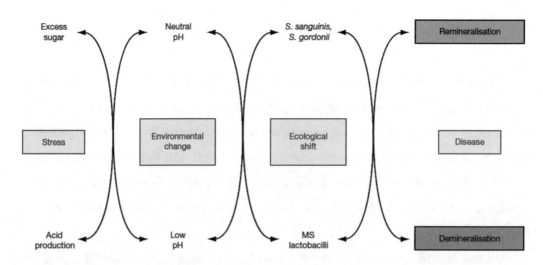

Figure 5.4   The ecological plaque hypothesis and the aetiology of dental caries

MS, mutans streptococci

Source: Marsh P. D., Nyvad B. (2008) In: Fejerskov O., Kidd E. *Dental Caries: The Disease and Its Clinical Management* (2nd edn.). Reproduced with permission of John Wiley & Sons, Inc.

(选自 *Dentistry at a Glance*, 1st Edition, Part 2, Chapter 32, Figure 32.4)

6. Summary

Understanding that caries occurs because of alterations in the ecology of the oral biofilm is important as it provides a clear theoretical basis for the preventive activities described in other parts of this book.

The importance of toothbrushing and the importance of sugar control are evidence based and biologically based.

Word List

1. juxtaposition [ˌdʒʌkstəpəˈzɪʃn] *n.* 并置；并列；毗邻；并排
2. demineralisation [ˌdemiːnrəlaɪˈzeɪʃən] *n.* 脱矿
3. remineralization [ˌremiːnrəlaɪˈzeɪʃn] *n.* 再矿化；去矿化作用
4. carbohydrate [ˌkɑːbəʊˈhaɪdreɪt] *n.* 碳水化合物；糖类
5. streptococcus [ˌstreptəˈkɒkəs] *n.* 链球菌属
6. actinomyces [ˌæktɪnəʊˈmaɪsiːz] *n.* 放线菌属

7. haemophilus [ˌhiːməˈfɪləs] *n.* 嗜血杆菌属

8. mutants streptococci [ˈmjuːtənts ˌstreptəˈkɒkaɪ] 变异链球菌

9. lactobacilus [ˌlæktəʊbəˈsɪləs] *n.* 乳杆菌属

10. anaerobic [ˌænəˈrəʊbɪk] *adj.* 厌氧的

11. glycoprotein [ˌglaɪkəʊˈprəʊtiːn] *n.* 糖蛋白

12. phosphoprotein [fɒsfəʊˈprəʊtiːn] *n.* 磷蛋白

13. porosity [pɔːˈrɒsəti] *n.* 多孔性

📝 Notes

❶ After a week of enamel being in juxtaposition with an undisturbed biofilm, although no changes would be seen clinically, microscopically the outer enamel surface can be seen to have signs of dissolution, making the enamel slightly more porous.

釉质表面的生物膜存在一周后，即使临床上看不到变化，但在显微镜下可以看到釉质外表面有溶解的迹象，从而使釉质形成多孔结构。

❷ As the bacterial deposits increase, the oxygen concentration lessens—thus plaque on teeth starts life composed of aerobic species but increasingly shifts to being made up of greater numbers of facultative anaerobes.

随着细菌沉积的增加，氧浓度降低，牙齿上的菌斑开始由需氧菌逐渐转变为主要由兼性厌氧菌组成。

❸ An active enamel lesion, or white-spot lesion, will have a chalky surface because the demineralisation and increased porosity cause loss of translucency.

因为脱矿和孔隙度增加导致釉质半透明性丧失，活跃的釉质龋损或龋白斑表面呈白垩色。

❹ It appears that bacteria are initially attracted to the tooth's pellicle by weak physicochemical forces but then adhesins on the cell wall interact with the pellicle.

细菌最初被微弱的物理化学力吸附到牙表面，但随后细菌细胞壁上的黏附分子直接与获得性膜发生相互作用。

（本单元由边专选编）

（文字部分选自 *Dentistry at a Glance*, 1st Edition, Part 2, Chapter 32）

Unit 6 ▶ Caries in Deciduous Teeth

1. Dental Caries

Dental caries is the localised destruction of susceptible dental hard tissue by acidic by-products from bacterial fermentation of dietary carbohydrates [1]. Therefore, it is a bacterial driven, site-specific, multifactorial dynamic disease process that is general, chronic and results from an imbalance in the physiological equilibrium between tooth mineral and plaque fluid [2].

The caries process is the dynamic sequence of biofilm-tooth interactions that can occur over time on and within a tooth surface. This process involves a shift in the balance between destructive factors (favouring demineralisation) and protective factors (favouring remineralisation). This disease process can be moderated, or even arrested, at any time by therapies that enhance the remineralisation process [3].

Primary teeth play a critical role in the growth and development of a child. In addition to their roles in aesthetics, mastication, speech, normal oral function and expected growth, another major function of the primary teeth is to provide space for their permanent successors until the permanent teeth erupt.

The condition of the primary dentition and the occlusal relationship of the maxillary teeth to the mandibular teeth directly influence both the functional and morphological development of the permanent dentition [4]. The primary teeth maintain the natural length of the dental arch and so permit the permanent teeth to erupt in an orderly fashion with adequate space. Some of the permanent teeth (premolars) are smaller than their primary predecessors while others are larger (permanent incisors and canines). Furthermore, the

---

本单元正文内容选自 Elizabeth Kay 所著 *Dentistry at a Glance*, John Wiley & Sons, Inc., 2016, Chapter 67, pp.140-141, 选用时图表序号有改动。

eruption pattern is not a uniform sequence. Therefore, without the primary teeth, the permanent successors can not assume their correct position in the dental arch.

2. Consequences of Leaving Untreated Carious Primary Teeth

The consequences of leaving dental caries in primary teeth untreated, which are illustrated in Figure 6.1, may include short-or long-term consequences or even rare sequelae.

2.1 Short Term

a. Pain

b. Infection, e.g., abscess, cellulitis

c. Emergency visits and possible hospitalization

d. Poor appetite

e. Disturbed sleep

f. Loss of days at school, kindergarten and playgroups with restricted activity and ability to play

g. Reduced ability to learn and concentrate at school

h. Need for tooth extraction

i. Need for treatment under general anaesthesia

j. Premature loss of primary molars predisposing to malocclusion in the permanent dentition

2.2 Long Term

a. Higher risk of new carious lesions in other primary teeth and the succeeding permanent dentition

b. Poor oral health and dental disease often continues into adulthood

c. Affect child's general health, resulting in insufficient physical development especially in height and weight

d. Increased treatment costs and time for parents

e. Potential adverse effects on speech, nutrition and quality of life

2.3 Rare Sequelae

a. Suborbital cellulitis

b. Unexplained recurrent fevers

c. Acute otitis media

d. abscess.

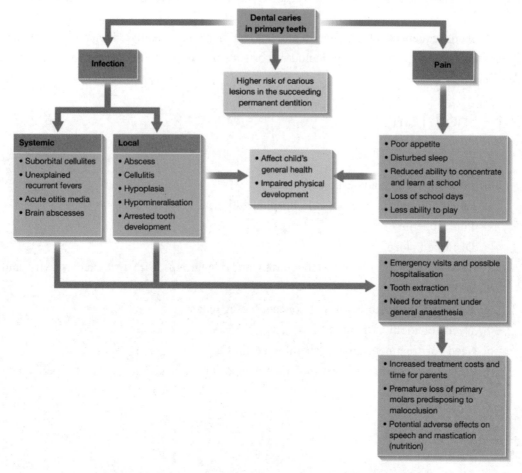

Figure 6.1　Consequences of carious lesions in the primary dentition

（选自 *Dentistry at a Glance*，1st Edition，Part 2，Chapter 67，Figure 67.1）

3.　Management of Carious Primary Teeth

3.1　Preventive Measures

Expectant mothers should be educated about：

a. The importance of nutrition throughout pregnancy

b. Good oral health and hygiene for themselves

c. Infant dietary habits

d. Early dental visits

e. Tooth brushing and fluoride preparations

f. The value of early dental check-ups for the child.

3.2　Fissure Sealants

These are recommended for primary and permanent molars in children with a history of dental caries and those who are in high-risk groups [5]. Fissure sealants have been proven to be effective; however, they need regular maintenance and repair.

3.3　Restorative Management

Prior to any definitive treatment plan the following factors must be considered:

a. Extent of the disease

b. Child's age and level of co-operation

c. Parents' attitude and motivation towards dental treatment.

3.4　Primary Anterior Teeth

The reason for restoring carious primary incisors and canines is to allow the child to retain these teeth, so as to allow natural exfoliation without any pulpal complications [6]. The treatment options available are:

a. Restorations with composite resin strip crowns, compomer, glass ionomer cements or stainless steel crowns

b. Pulp therapy (pulpotomy or pulpectomy)

c. Extraction.

3.5　Primary Molars

Depending on the extent of a carious lesion, one of the following materials can be used for the restoration of primary molars.

a. Composite resin

b. Compomer

c. Stainless steel crowns

d. Glass ionomer cement

e. Amalgam

f. Pulp therapy（pulpotomy or pulpectomy）

g. Extraction.

3.6   Space Maintainers

Premature loss of primary teeth by extraction can have an influence on the occlusion and space for the teeth of the permanent dentition. Very rarely it is thought necessary to use space maintaining appliances in an attempt to retain the space for the succeeding permanent teeth. Numerous factors, such as the age of the patient, teeth present, caries status, level of oral hygiene, the willingness of the parents to bring the child for treatment and the patient to accept the treatment, need to be considered prior to deciding to insert a space maintainer [7].

📋 Word List

1. caries [ˈkeəriːz] *n.* 龋齿

2. deciduous teeth（primary teeth）乳牙

3. susceptible [səˈseptəbl] *adj.* 易感的

4. bacterial [bækˈtɪrɪəl] *adj.* 细菌的

5. fermentation [ˌfɜːmenˈteɪʃn] *n.* 发酵

6. equilibrium [ˌiːkwɪˈlɪbrɪəm] *n.* 平衡

7. plaque [plæk] *n.* 牙菌斑

8. aesthetics [esˈθetɪks] *n.* 美观；美学

9. mastication [ˌmæstɪˈkeɪʃn] *n.* 咀嚼

10. permanent teeth 恒牙

11. erupt [ɪˈrʌpt] *v.* 萌出

12. morphological [ˌmɔːfəˈlɒdʒɪkl] *adj.* 形态学的

13. incisor [ɪnˈsaɪzə(r)] *n.* 切牙；门牙

14. predecessor [ˈpredəsesə(r)] *n.* 前身；（被取代的）原有事物

15. sequelae [sɪˈkwiːliː] *n.* 并发症（sequela 的复数）；后遗症

16. abscess [ˈæbses] *n.* 脓肿；脓疮

17. cellulitis [ˌseljuˈlaɪtɪs] *n.* 蜂窝组织炎

18. hospitalisation [ˌhɒspɪtəlaɪˈzeɪʃn] *n.* 住院治疗

19. appetite [ˈæpɪtaɪt] *n.* 胃口；食欲

20. extraction [ɪkˈstrækʃn] *n.* (牙齿)拔除；取出

21. general anaesthesia 全身麻醉

22. premature loss (牙齿)早失

23. malocclusion [ˌmæləˈkluːʒən] *n.* 错𬌗畸形

24. suborbital [sʌbˈɔːbɪtəl] *adj.* 眶下的

25. otitis media 中耳炎

26. pregnancy [ˈpregnənsɪ] *n.* 孕期；妊娠期

27. hygiene [ˈhaɪdʒiːn] *n.* 卫生

28. fluoride [ˈflɔːraɪd] *n.* 氟化物

29. fissure sealants 窝沟封闭

30. restorative [rɪˈstɔːrətɪv] *adj.* 整形的；修复性的

31. composite resin strip crowns 复合树脂剥脱冠

32. compomer [kəmˈpəumə] *n.*(复合树脂与离子)复合体

33. glass ionomer cements 玻璃离子水门汀

34. stainless steel crowns 不锈钢金属冠(金属预成冠)

35. pulpotomy [pʌlˈpɔtəmi] *n.* 牙髓切断术

36. pulpectomy [pʌlˈpektəmɪ] *n.* 去髓术；牙髓摘除术

37. amalgam [əˈmælgəm] *n.* 汞合金

38. space maintainers 间隙保持器

📝 Notes

❶ Dental caries is the localised destruction of susceptible dental hard tissue by acidic by-products from bacterial fermentation of dietary carbohydrates.
龋病是细菌发酵食物中的碳水化合物产生的酸性副产物，由易感牙体硬组织的局部破坏产生。

❷ Therefore，it is a bacterial driven，site-specific，multifactorial dynamic disease process that is general，chronic and results from an imbalance in the physiological equilibrium between tooth mineral and plaque fluid.

因此，它(龋病)是一种由细菌驱动、部位特异、多因素的疾病，是一种具有普遍性、慢性进行性的疾病过程，是牙体矿物质和牙菌斑液之间生理平衡失调的结果。

❸ This disease process can be moderated, or even arrested, at any time by therapies that enhance the remineralisation process.
这种疾病进程可以在任何时候通过增强牙齿再矿化过程的治疗而减缓，或甚至停止。

❹ The condition of the primary dentition and the occlusal relationship of the maxillary teeth to the mandibular teeth directly influence both the functional and morphological development of the permanent dentition.
乳牙列的状况、上下颌牙齿的咬合关系直接影响恒牙列的功能和形态发育。

❺ These are recommended for primary and permanent molars in children with a history of dental caries and those who are in high-risk groups.
有龋病史的儿童和高龋风险人群的乳恒磨牙推荐进行窝沟封闭。

❻ The reason for restoring carious primary incisors and canines is to allow the child to retain these teeth, so as to allow natural exfoliation without any pulpal complications.
修复龋损乳切牙及乳尖牙是为了让孩子保留这些牙齿，从而在没有任何牙髓并发症的情况下自然脱落。

❼ Numerous factors, such as the age of the patient, teeth present, caries status, level of oral hygiene, the willingness of the parents to bring the child for treatment and the patient to accept the treatment, need to be considered prior to deciding to insert a space maintainer.
在决定戴入间隙保持器之前，需要考虑许多因素，例如患者的年龄、存留的牙齿、龋齿状况、口腔卫生水平、父母带孩子去治疗的意愿以及患儿接受治疗的意愿。

(本单元由何淼选编)

(文字部分选自 *Dentistry at a Glance*, 1st Edition, Part 2, Chapter 67)

Unit 7 ▶ Tooth Isolation

1. Reasons for Tooth Isolation

In restorative dentistry teeth are isolated for the following several reasons:

a. **To improve patient's comfort and safety** : Saliva as well as the water produced by handpieces and 3-in-1 syringes can accumulate and cause discomfort. Some of the chemicals and liquids used during operative work can be harmful to the soft tissue and cause irritation or burns. Also small and sharp instruments (for example, endodontic files and reamers) can dislodge, putting the patient at the risk of inhaling the implement.

b. **Improvement of access and visibility** . Constant water spray from the handpiece topped up by saliva can reduce visibility dramatically.

c. **Prevention of contamination of the restorative procedure** . Several species of microorganisms inhabit the oral cavity. These microorganisms can contaminate the prepared cavities and pulpal tissues and lead to new or persistent infections.

d. **Allowing for proper placement of restorative materials** . Liquid contamination can have a negative effect on the mechanical properties of almost all of the direct restorative materials. When adhesive materials are used, any liquid contamination can cause failure of the restoration.

2. Tooth Isolation Techniques

There are several techniques that can be used to isolate a tooth. Some of the most

本单元正文内容选自 Elizabeth Kay 所著 *Dentistry at a Glance*, John Wiley & Sons, Inc., 2016, Chapter 40, pp. 90-91. 选用时删减原文部分图片,图片序号有改动,文字内容有少量改动。

commonly used techniques are described in this part.

2.1   Aspiration

A **high-volume suction tip** (Figure 7.1a) can be used by the dental assistant to remove the excess fluid from the operative field. This is an effective device to remove large quantities of fluid quickly.

Additionally, the **Saliva ejector** is also a useful tool to remove fluids from the oral cavity (Figure 7.1b). It can be a very helpful as an adjunctive tool to be used while a rubber dam is in place to improve the patient's comfort [1].

A **Svedopter** (**flange**) is used to isolate the lower teeth. It retracts the tongue and aspirates fluids at the same time. By adding cotton wool rolls on the buccal aspect, enough isolation can be achieved for impression taking or cementation [2].

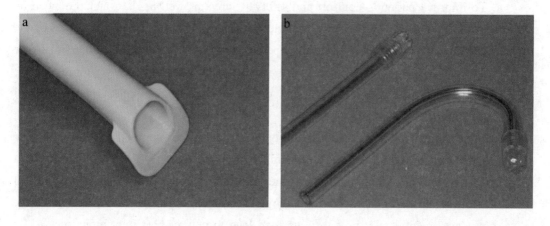

Figure 7.1

(a) High volume suction tip and (b) saliva ejector; saliva ejectors can be moulded for optimal fit.

(选自 *Dentistry at a Glance*, 1st Edition, Part 2, Chapter 40, Figure 40.1)

2.2   Cotton Wool Rolls and Cellulose Pads

Cotton wools rolls are used to absorb fluids and retract the lips or cheeks. They can provide an adequate dry field when used in conjunction with effective aspiration. When placed in the buccal or labial sulcus, a mirror can be used to keep the cotton wool roll in place [3] (Figure 7.2). **Cellulose pads** are placed on the buccal sulcus and can be used to absorb moisture from the parotid duct.

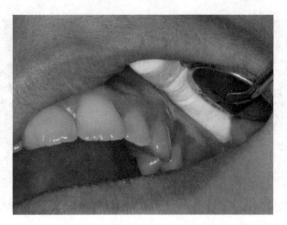

Figure 7.2

Cotton wool roll placed in the buccal sulcus; a mirror can be used to keep the cotton wool roll in place.

（选自 *Dentistry at a Glance*, 1st Edition, Part 2, Chapter 40, Figure 40.3）

2.3 Rubber Dam

Rubber dam was introduced to the dental profession in 1864 and has remained the gold standard for tooth isolation [4]. The dam material is available in variety of colours. In restorative dentistry it is important to choose a colour that contrasts with the colour of the teeth.

1. **Material**. The dam material is available in several thicknesses or gauges. For restorative work, heavy and extra heavy gauges (0.15-0.35 mm) are recommended. They apply as easily as thinner dams but are less likely to tear. They are available in latex and latex-free forms.

2. **Clamps**. Rubber dam clamps are the usual means of securing the dam. There are three basic types of clamps available (Figure 7.3). The dam can be placed on a winged-clamp prior to the application (Figure 7.4). When using a wingless clamp, rubber dam can be placed in the mouth prior or after placement of the clamp. The butterfly clamp serves as a gingival retractor at the same time as retaining the rubber dam in situ [5]. Clamps are available in different sizes. When choosing a clamp, it is important that only its jaw points contact the tooth. This will create a four-point contact.

3. **Floss ligatures**. It is widely recommended that dental floss should be attached to every clamp used in the mouth. This allows retrieval of the clamp if the clamp dislodges or breaks. Certainly it is wise to attach floss to the dam if it is placed in the mouth prior to the application of the clamp; however, the floss can cause leakage and therefore once the

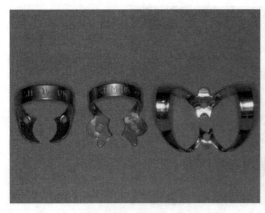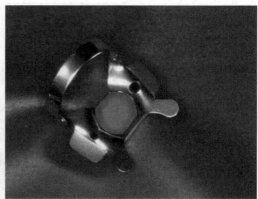

Figure 7.3　(left)　　　　　　　　　　　　　Figure 7.4　(right)

Clamps, from left to right: wingless, winged and butterfly.

（选自 *Dentistry at a Glance*, 1st Edition, Part 2, Chapter 40,Figure 40.5）

Note the wings underneath the dam; this complex can now be delivered into the mouth.

（选自 *Dentistry at a Glance*, 1st Edition, Part 2, Chapter 40,Figure 40.6）

rubber dam application is finished, the floss should be removed [6]. Of course if the clamp fractures or dislodges after the application is finished, the dam will prevent dislodgement of the clamp into the oral cavity. When a winged-clamp is attached to the dam prior to placement of the clamp onto a tooth, the use of floss ligature is unnecessary.

4. **Placement**. Teeth should be cleaned, if necessary, and contacts should be checked with floss to ensure the dam can pass the contacts with ease [7]. If occlusal restorations are planned, the occlusion should be marked prior to the rubber dam application. A rubber dam stamp can be used to locate the position of the teeth. When doing restorative work on a posterior tooth, usually the most distal tooth in that quadrant is clamped. This will allow exposure of several teeth. Using a rubber dam punch, holes of varying sizes will be created according to the size of the corresponding teeth (Figure 7.5). If a winged-clamp is used, the dam will be attached to the clamp. This combination will then be transferred into the mouth. If a wingless clamp is used, the clamp is placed on the tooth first. The dam is then stretched to pass over the clamp and wraps around the neck of the tooth. A waxed floss is recommended to floss the dam through the interproximal contacts.

5. **Inversion of the dam**. The dam should be inverted around the neck of the teeth. If the dam is directed occlusally, fluids will push through to the operative field. High-volume air is used to dry the teeth and dam surface to facilitate inversion. A No. 23 explorer or a No.1-2 plastic instrument can be used to invert the dam (Figure 7.6).

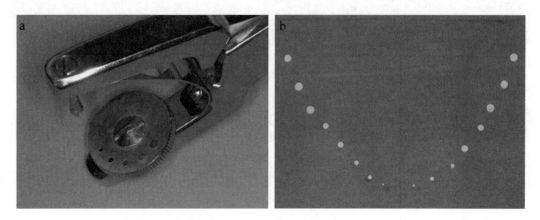

Figure 7.5

Using the punch (a) holes in varying sizes can be created (b), corresponding to the differences in the sizes of the teeth.

(选自 *Dentistry at a Glance*, 1st Edition, Part 2, Chapter 40, Figure 40.7)

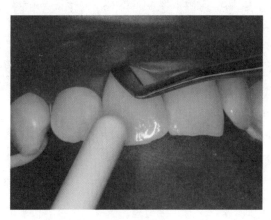

Figure 7.6

The dam is inverted using a flat plastic instrument; note that the assistant can facilitate this by blowing air at high pressure.

(选自 *Dentistry at a Glance*, 1st Edition, Part 2, Chapter 40, Figure 40.9)

📑 Word List

1. isolation [ˌaɪsəˈleɪʃn] *n.* 隔离；孤立；绝缘
2. restorative dentistry [医] 牙科修复学
3. handpiece [hænd'piːs] *n.* 牙科手机

4. irritation [ˌɪrɪˈteɪʃn] n. (身体某部位的)疼痛；刺激(作用)

5. syringe [sɪˈrɪndʒ] n. 注射器；注射筒；灌肠器；注油筒；洗涤器

6. endodontic files 根管锉

7. reamer [ˈriːmə(r)] n. [机]铰刀；钻孔器

8. put...at the risk of 把……置于风险中

9. dislodge [dɪsˈlɒdʒ] vt. 把……逐出；驱逐；vi. 移走；离开原位

10. inhaling [ɪnˈheɪlɪŋ] v. 吸入(inhale 的现在分词)

11. dramatically [drəˈmætɪklɪ] adv. 戏剧地；显著地

12. contamination [kənˌtæmɪˈneɪʃn] n. 污染

13. microorganism [ˌmaɪkrəʊˈɔːɡənɪzəm] n. [微]微生物

14. pulpal [ˈpʌlp(ə)l] adj. 牙髓的

15. adhesive [ədˈhiːsɪv] adj. 黏着的；有黏性的 n. 黏着剂；胶水

16. aspiration [ˌæspəˈreɪʃn] n. 抱负；志向；[医]吸引术；抽吸

17. suction [ˈsʌkʃn] n. 吸；抽吸；吸出；相吸

18. saliva ejector 吸唾器

19. adjunctive [əˈdʒʌŋktɪv] adj. 附属的；附加的

20. flange [flændʒ] n. (机械等的)凸缘；(火车的)轮缘

21. retract [rɪˈtrækt] vt. & vi. 撤回或撤消；缩回；缩进

22. aspirate [ˈæspərət] v. 吸气；n. 送气音

23. impression taking 取模

24. cementation [ˌsiːmenˈteɪʃn] n. 黏固；烧结

25. sulcus [ˈsʌlkəs] n. 沟；槽；裂缝

26. cellulose [ˈseljuləʊs] n. 纤维素

27. labial sulcus 唇沟

28. moisture [ˈmɒɪstʃə] n. 水分；湿气；潮湿；降雨量

29. parotid duct 腮腺导管

30. rubber dam 橡皮障

31. gauge [ɡeɪdʒ] n. 测量的标准或范围；尺度；标准；测量仪器；评估

32. latex [ˈleɪteks] n. 乳胶；(尤指橡胶树的)橡浆

33. in situ [ˌɪn ˈsaɪtuː] 在原位置；在原处

34. floss [flɒs] n. 牙线；vi. 用牙线清洁牙齿

35. ligature [ˈlɪɡətʃə(r)] n. (用于紧缚的)带子；绳索；绷带 v. 结扎

36. rubber dam clamp 橡皮障夹

37. gingival [dʒɪnˈdʒaɪvəl] adj. 牙龈的

38. jaw [dʒɔː] *n.* 颌；颚
39. retrieval [rɪˈtriːvl] *n.* 收回；挽回；检索
40. quadrant [ˈkwɒdrənt] *n.* 四分之一圆
41. rubber dam punch 橡皮障打孔器
42. stretched to 拉伸到
43. waxed floss [医]有蜡牙线
44. occlusal [əˈkluːs(ə)l] *adj.* 咬合面的
45. interproximal [ˌɪntəˈprɒksɪməl] *adj.* 邻间的
46. inversion [ɪnˈvɜːʒn] *n.* 倒置

📝 Notes

❶ It can be a very helpful as an adjunctive tool to be used while a rubber dam is in place to improve the patient's comfort.
在使用橡皮障时，它可以作为一个辅助工具，以提高患者的舒适度。

❷ By adding cotton wool rolls on the buccal aspect, enough isolation can be achieved for impression taking or cementation.
在颊侧放置棉卷能够为印模或粘接操作提供足够的隔离。

❸ When placed in the buccal or labial sulcus, a mirror can be used to keep the cotton wool roll in place.
当棉球卷放置于颊沟或唇沟内时，可以使用口镜保持其固定在原位。

❹ Rubber dam was introduced to the dental profession in 1864 and has remained the gold standard for tooth isolation.
橡皮障于 1864 年被引入牙科行业，一直是牙齿隔离的金标准。

❺ The butterfly clamp serves as a gingival retractor at the same time as retaining the rubber dam in situ.
蝴蝶夹同时充当牙龈牵引器，并保持橡皮障就位。

❻ Certainly it is wise to attach floss to the dam if it is placed in the mouth prior to the application of the clamp; however, the floss can cause leakage and therefore once the rubber dam application is finished, the floss should be removed.

当然，在安装橡皮障夹之前将牙线系在橡皮障上是明智之举；然而，牙线可能会造成渗漏，因此一旦橡皮障放置完毕，应将牙线移除。

❼ Teeth should be cleaned, if necessary, and contacts should be checked with floss to ensure the dam can pass the contacts with ease.

如有必要应清洁牙齿，并使用牙线检查牙齿邻接点，以确保橡皮障能轻松通过邻接点。

（本单元由边专、孟柳燕选编）

（文字部分选自 *Dentistry at a Glance*, 1st Edition, Part 2, Chapter 40）

Unit 8 ▸ Cavity Preparation for Plastic Tooth Restorations

The decision to restore a tooth must be taken carefully, and only when the caries in the tooth has progressed to a stage where remineralization and repair can no longer be expected. All restorations are 'temporary' in as much as all will progress to more severe lesions eventually, if the patient can not maintain a good oral hygiene.

The principles that underpin cavity preparation were first established by G.V. Black and are just as valid today as they were in 19th century (Figure 8.1). Essentially, these translate as:

a. Gain access to the decay (when the caries is through an enamel surface).

b. Remove the caries and resulting unsupported enamel.

c. Assess which restorative material will give the 'best' outcome and bearing in mind the properties of the material.

d. Modify the residual tooth tissue to make a cavity that will maximise the life expectancy of the restorative material.

1. Accessing Caries

Caries progression through enamel into dentine results in destruction in the dentine that is much 'wider' than the damage to the enamel. Thus it is necessary to remove some of the sound but unsupported enamel to gain adequate access to the underlying carious dentine and obtain an interface with sufficient mechanical strength. Enamel is the hardest of all tissues in the body and requires very powerful cutting tools to remove it. There are a number of options available to the dentist, including air abrasion and lasers, but the most common is a tungsten carbide tipped or diamond-coated bur in a dental handpiece, most

---

本单元正文内容选自 Elizabeth Kay 所著 *Dentistry at a Glance*, John Wiley & Sons, Inc., 2016, Chapter 43, pp.96-97, 选用时文字内容有少量变动,图片序号有改动。

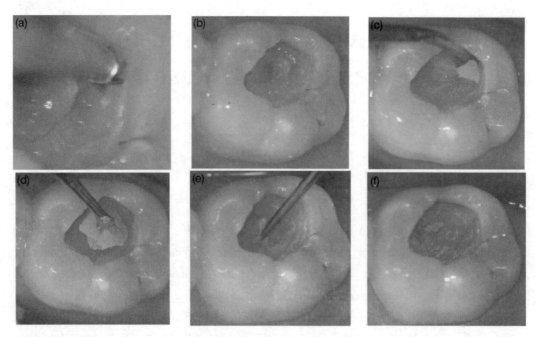

Figure 8.1

The current clinical practice of mechanical excavation combines a peripheral dentine excavation, carried out using a round burr (a, b), with elimination of the centrally infected tissue using an excavator (c, d). The probe is used to assess clinical consistency, and here dentine that is hard to the touch has not yet been obtained (e). Note that the deeper and soft carious dentine is a fragmented tissue (f). An excavation close to the pulp represents a risk because cracks along the fragments may lead to pulp exposure.

Source: Kidd E.A.M. et al. (2008) In: Fejerskov O., Kidd E. *Dental Caries: The Disease and Its Clinical Management* (2nd edn.). Reproduced with permission of John Wiley & Sons, Inc.

(选自 *Dentistry at a Glance*, 1st Edition, Part 2, Chapter 43, Figure 43.1)

commonly an air rotor [1]. The initial approach into the carious lesion should be sufficient to allow access to the decay whist keeping the cavity small to prevent unnecessary removal of sound tooth tissue.

Once you have exposed the carious you need to remove the carious tissue.

Tip: Make your initial access into a carious lesion using a bur with a cutting tip no more than 2 mm long to reduce the risk of exposing the pulp. You can use the length of the cutting surface of the bur as a depth guide.

2. Caries Removal

We now recognize that there are multiple 'levels' to a carious dentine lesion. The most important distinction from a clinical perspective is the differentiation between caries-infected and caries-affected dentine. Caries is essentially a process of demineralization driven by acid-producing bacteria. As the caries progresses through dentine the acids cause demineralization and the demineralized dentine is subsequently colonised by bacteria. So:

a. The carious dentine closer to the enamel will be both demineralized and infected with bacteria, this is the caries-infected dentine and should be removed.

b. The carious dentine closer to the pulp may (depending on the extent of the lesion) be demineralized without infection, this is caries-affected dentine and can be left during cavity preparation depending on the choice of restorative material.

c. Differentiating between infected and affected dentine during cavity preparation can be difficult.

2.1 Texture

There are subtle changes in texture between the two; all carious dentine will be relatively soft, wet and crumbly but caries-infected dentine will be softer and wetter than caries-affected tissue. Indeed, caries-affected dentine will become progressively harder as you progress closer to the advancing margin of the carious lesion, also called leathery dentine [2]. Soft dentine can be removed with a bur, preferably in a slow handpiece or using excavators, but the operator needs considerable experience to differentiate between the subtle texture differences in dentine (Figure 8.2). The most common advice is to remove all wet crumbly (friable) dentine during this process.

Tip: Wherever possible practice removing caries on extracted human teeth to try to develop the sense of feel for carious dentine.

2.2 Bacterial Presence

A variety of dyes have been advocated to try to differentiate between the presence and absence of bacteria (and hence infected and affected dentine). However, it is now recognized that while these dyes may be an adjunct; they are not selective solely for bacteria, but rather staining the demineralized matrix of carious dentine and other areas of dentine with reduced mineralization such as the amelodentinal junction and circum-pulpal dentine [3].

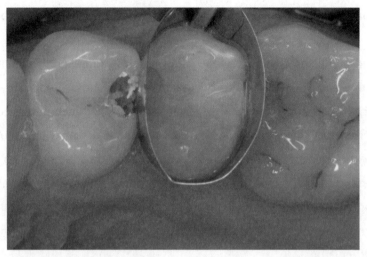

Figure 8.2   Partially excavated cavity; note the soft, wet dentine.

Source: van Amerongen J. P. et al. (2008) In: Fejerskov O., Kidd E. *Dental Caries: The Disease and Its Clinical Management* (2nd edn.). Reproduced with permission of John Wiley & Sons, Inc.

(选自 *Dentistry at a Glance*, 1st Edition, Part 2,Chapter 43,Figure 43.2)

2.3   Chemomechanical Caries Removal

A mixture of sodium hypochlorite with lysine, leucine and glutamic acids, and some other amino acids in a carboxymethyl cellulose base is commercially available as Carisolv®. Activating this product results in the formation of N-monochloroglycine and N-monochloroaminobutyric acid. When these are applied to carious dentine they dissolve the collagen in the carious lesion making the infected dentine easier to remove. Recent evidence suggests that dentine removal guided by Carisolve is probably the most reliable method for removing infected dentine and leaving the affected dentine that can then remineralize.

3.   Unsupported Enamel

Enamel is a brittle material and needs to be supported by dentine to exhibit durability. Where dentine is destroyed by caries, eliminating support for the enamel, consideration needs to be given to removing the enamel.

If unsupported enamel is not removed it can fracture during or after restoration of the tooth with resulting marginal discrepancies around an amalgam restoration and marginal gaps round a composite that may result in postoperative sensitivity [4].

Tip：When in doubt about the support for remaining enamel, push firmly against the enamel with an amalgam plugger in all directions.

📑 Word List

1. tungsten [ˈtʌŋstən] *n.* 钨
2. crumbly [ˈkrʌmblɪ] *n.* 易碎的
3. carboxymethyl [kɑːbɒkˈsiːmeθɪl] *n.* 羧甲基
4. excavation [ˌekskəˈveɪʃn] *v.* 挖掘
5. glutamic acid [gluːˈtæmɪk ˈæsɪd] 谷氨酸
6. hypochlorite [ˌhaɪpəˈklɔːraɪt] *n.* 次氯酸盐
7. hygiene [ˈhaɪdʒiːn] *n.* 卫生；保健
8. lysine [ˈlaɪsiːn] *n.* 赖氨酸
9. leucine [ˈluːsiːn] *n.* 亮氨酸
10. underpin [ˌʌndəˈpɪn] *v.* 支撑；加强；构成

✍ Notes

❶ There are a number of options available to the dentist, including air abrasion and lasers, but the most common is a tungsten carbide tipped or diamond-coated bur in a dental handpiece, most commonly an air rotor.
牙医有很多工具可选，包括空气喷砂和激光技术，但最常用的还是通过空气马达驱动连接在牙科手机上的碳钨钢或是金刚石车针。

❷ All carious dentine will be relatively soft, wet and crumbly but caries-infected dentine will be softer and wetter than caries-affected tissue. Indeed, caries-affected dentine will become progressively harder as you progress closer to the advancing margin of the carious lesion, also called leathery dentine.
所有龋坏牙本质都相对较软、潮湿和易碎，但龋感染牙本质比龋损牙本质更软、

更潮湿。事实上，龋损牙本质距离龋坏进展边缘越近越坚硬，称为皮革样牙本质。

❸ However, it is now recognized that while these dyes may be an adjunct; they are not selective solely for bacteria, but rather staining the demineralized matrix of carious dentine and other areas of dentine with reduced mineralization such as the amelodentinal junction and circum-pulpal dentine.

虽然认为这些染料可以辅助辨别龋坏，但它们不仅只着色细菌，对龋坏牙本质的脱矿基质和矿化较弱的釉牙本质界以及牙髓周围的牙本质也能染色。

❹ If unsupported enamel is not removed it can fracture during or after restoration of the tooth with resulting marginal discrepancies around an amalgam restoration and marginal gaps round a composite that may result in postoperative sensitivity.

如果无基釉未被去除，它可能在牙齿修复期间或之后破裂，导致汞合金修复体周围与牙齿的边缘不密合以及复合材料周围的边缘间隙，这可能导致术后牙齿敏感。

（本单元由边专选编）
（文字部分选自 *Dentistry at a Glance*, 1st Edition, Part 2, Chapter 43）

Unit 9 ▶ Choice of Plastic Restorative Materials

Filling cavities is a crucial step in restoring the function and aesthetics of the tooth [1]. Selection of an appropriate restorative material will depend on a variety of factors:

a. The tooth concerned (and hence the need for an aesthetic material) along with the location of the cavity on the tooth.

b. The extent of destruction of tooth tissue (and hence the physical characteristics of the restorative material in terms of durability).

c. The amount of remaining tooth tissue (which can be used to support/retain the new restoration).

d. The caries risk status of the individual.

e. The ability to attain a required level of moisture control to maximize the chances of restoration longevity.

1. Location of the Tooth and Extent of the Cavity

Generally, teeth in the anterior region of the mouth will be restored using tooth-coloured materials while the options for posterior teeth include metallic restorations where aesthetics may not be so critical [2].

1.1 Anterior Teeth

There are two major groups of tooth-coloured direct restorative materials: glass ionomer cements (GICs) and dental composite resins. Their relative longevity can be

---

本单元正文内容选自 Elizabeth Kay 所著 *Dentistry at a Glance*, John Wiley & Sons, Inc., 2016, Chapter 44, pp.98-99, 选用时文字内容有少量变动,图表序号有改动。

compared in Figure 9.

　　Generally, the better aesthetic characteristics of composite resins predicate their use for the majority of anterior restorations, particularly extensive restorations involving the incisal edge of teeth. GICs are more likely to be used for small class III and class V restorations, particularly where the patient exhibits high caries risk.

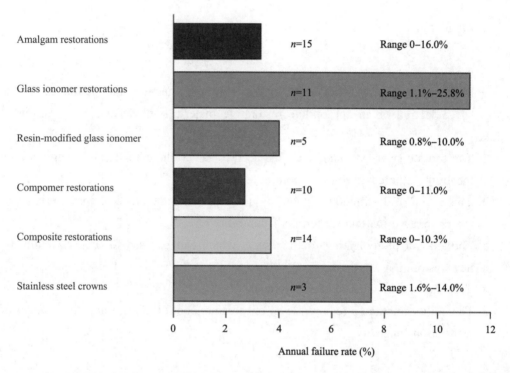

Figure 9

Median values and ranges for annual failure rates obtained in longitudinal studies of class I/II restorations in posterior primary teeth using different types of restorative materials; n, number of studies.

Source: Qvist V. (2008) In: Fejerskov O., Kidd E. *Dental Caries: The Disease and Its Clinical Management* (2nd edn). Reproduced with permission of John Wiley & Sons, Inc.

（选自 *Dentistry at a Glance*, 1st Edition, Part 2, Chapter 44, Figure 44.1）

1.2　Posterior Teeth

　　The choice of materials for posterior teeth includes not only composite resins and GICs but also includes dental amalgam [3]. Generally, GICs may be used for class V cavities and provisional restorations. The choice between composite resin and dental amalgam for load-bearing restorations on occlusal and proximal surfaces needs to be based on careful consideration of the following variables:

    a. **Extent of the cavity** : Dental amalgam exhibits greater longevity than composite resins with large restorations where wear of the composite in function becomes a significant problem.

    b. **Patient choice** : Some patients elect to have tooth-coloured restorations rather than metallic.

    c. **Hypersensitivity** : Some patients manifest a hypersensitivity reaction to dental amalgam with 'lichenoid eruptions' on the cheek mucosa proximate to the restorative material.

It is the responsibility of the dentist/ therapist to obtain informed consent from their patient concerning the choice of restorative material, and particularly when a composite resin is being used in a large cavity to explain that the restoration will exhibit reduced longevity compared with a dental amalgam restoration in the same cavity. There is an impending move to ban the use of dental amalgam to reduce the bio-availability of mercury in the environment. If this happens then the choices will be fewer unless new materials become available.

2. Quantity and Quality of Remaining Tooth Tissue

Restorations need to be both supported and retained by the remaining tooth tissue after cavity preparation. As a consequence, the amount of remaining tooth and its location influences the choice of restorative material. When there are substantial amounts of remaining tooth, there tend to be more options in terms of choice of material. As the amount of remaining tooth diminishes, the options reduce and restorations become bigger, favouring dental amalgam over composite resin in terms of durability. Perversely, with extreme loss of tooth tissue, where an adhesive approach to retention is the only possibility, composite resin may offer the best available alternative, as adhesive options with dental amalgam are not as effective as those for resin composite.

3. Caries Risk

There is limited evidence that GIC restorations are prone to the development of fewer carious lesions associated with the restoration than composite resin in high caries risk patients.

4. Moisture Control

Any restorative technique that is using an adhesive approach to retaining the restoration requires a high level of moisture control during restoration placement [4]. If either a dentine or an enamel surface that has been prepared for bonding is contaminated with saliva or blood a protein film forms on the surface of the tooth, preventing the formation of an acceptable adhesive bond. This applies to both GICs and resin composites. Contamination of the tooth surface will both reduce retention of the restoration and increase the risks of marginal leakage. This is probably the biggest single challenge to finding a replacement for dental amalgam.

5. Physical (Mechanical) Retention

Dental amalgam has no intrinsic capacity to bond to tooth tissue [5]. There are some techniques that can result in a bonded amalgam restoration but the majority of amalgam restorations are retained as a result of mechanical retention within a cavity. The nature of the carious process with spread of demineralisation along the amelodentinal junction (ADJ) results in cavities that are wider at the base than the top, making a naturally undercut shape. The extent of undercut needs to be reassessed once unsupported enamel has been removed to ensure there is adequate mechanical retention present.

Where there is extensive loss of tooth tissue involving the cusps of a tooth, there may be the need to prepare grooves or pits in the remaining dentine to develop mechanical retention for the cavity. These are often used in association with a bonded approach to maximize the retention of the amalgam in a tooth.

📑 Word List

1. composite resin ['kɒmpəzɪt 'rezɪn] 复合树脂
2. hypersensitivity [ˌhaɪpəˌsensə'tɪvətɪ] n. 高敏感度
3. dental amalgam ['dentl ə'mælgəm] 牙科银汞合金
4. amelodentinal junction [ˌæmeləʊ'dentɪnəl 'dʒʌŋkʃn] 釉牙本质界
5. cavity ['kævətɪ] n. 窝洞
6. aesthetic [es'θetɪk] n. 美学

7. glass ionomer cement [glɑːs ˈaɪɒnəmə sɪˈment] 玻璃离子粘固剂
8. metallic restoration [məˈtælɪk ˌrestəˈreɪʃn] 金属修复材料
9. caries risk [ˈkeəriːz rɪsk] 龋病风险
10. physical retention [ˈfɪzɪkl rɪˈtenʃn] 机械固位
11. undercut [ˌʌndəˈkʌt] n. 倒凹

📝 Notes

❶ Filling cavities is a crucial step in restoring the function and aesthetics of the tooth.
窝洞填充是恢复牙齿功能和美观的关键一步。

❷ Generally, teeth in the anterior region of the mouth will be restored using tooth-coloured materials while the options for posterior teeth include metallic restorations where aesthetics may not be so critical.
一般来说，前牙需要使用与牙齿相同颜色的材料进行修复，而后牙因为不需要过分考虑美观性，修复材料的选择会更多，比如可以考虑金属修复材料。

❸ The choice of materials for posterior teeth includes not only composite resins and GICs but also includes dental amalgam.
适用于后牙的充填材料不仅包括复合树脂和玻璃离子，还包括牙科银汞合金。

❹ Any restorative technique that is using an adhesive approach to retaining the restoration requires a high level of moisture control during restoration placement.
任何使用粘接方法为填充材料提供固位的临床操作都要求在填充过程中进行严格的隔湿。

❺ Dental amalgam has no intrinsic capacity to bond to tooth tissue.
牙科银汞合金与牙体组织没有任何粘合能力。

（本单元由尹伟选编）
（文字部分选自 *Dentistry at a Glance*, 1st Edition, Part 2, Chapter 44）

Unit 10 ▶ Pulp Therapy (Deciduous Teeth)

1. Introduction

The aim of pulp therapy in deciduous teeth is to remove inflamed pulp tissue, conserve the damaged tooth and restore function until the permanent successor erupts [1]. The main reason for the pulp of a tooth to become inflamed or infected is dental caries. It is important to take an accurate pain history in order to determine the level of pulp involvement and preoperative radiographs are useful to assess the extent of the carious lesion and its proximity to the pulp. Once caries has been removed from the tooth, it is easier to assess the level of pulpal exposure. Blood will be present at the exposure site if the pulp tissue is still vital.

Signs that may indicate pulp treatment is necessary are：

a. Occlusal caries extending into the pulpal tissue (usually 4 mm or more in depth).

b. Proximal caries extending into the marginal ridge.

c. Tooth mobility.

d. Sinus formation.

e. Furcation radiolucency on radiograph.

Symptoms that may indicate pulp treatment is necessary are：

a. Reversible pulpitis pain-pain on stimulus.

b. Irreversible pulpitis pain-pain is spontaneous and lasts.

c. Swelling.

There are various treatment options for deciduous teeth with pulpal involvement：

a. Indirect pulp capping.

本单元正文内容选自 Elizabeth Kay 所著 *Dentistry at a Glance*, John Wiley & Sons, Inc., 2016, Chapter 60, pp.126-127. 选用时表格有删除,图片序号有改动。

b. Vital pulpotomy.

c. Non-vital pulpotomy (desensitising).

d. Pulpectomy.

2. Indirect Pulp Capping

The purpose of this technique is to maintain pulp vitality by placing a lining onto deep dentin in order to eliminate bacteria and to stimulate secondary dentin.

2.1 Indications

a. An otherwise healthy mouth, similar to that shown in Figure 10.1a-c

b. Minor reversible pulpitis symptoms, e.g. pain on a stimulus only.

c. Deep caries but no abscess or swelling.

d. Caries not extending into pulp, so no pulpal exposure (Figure 10.2a).

2.2 Contraindications

a. Extensive caries into the pulp

b. Irreversible pulpitis symptoms, e.g., pain waking child at night or pain that lingers without a stimulus [2].

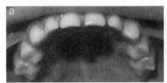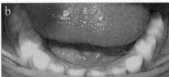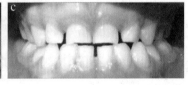

Figure 10.1

A healthy deciduous (a) upper arch, (b) lower arch and (c) dentition.

(选自 *Dentistry at a Glance*, 1st Edition, Part 2, Chapter 60, Figure 60.1)

3. Vital Pulpotomy

This procedure involves removing the coronal pulp that is inflamed and infected (Figure 10.2b), leaving healthy radicular pulp. The coronal pulp will bleed as it is still vital.

a.　　　　　　　　　　　b.　　　　　　　　　　　c.

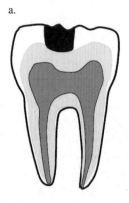 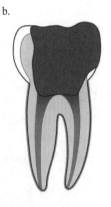 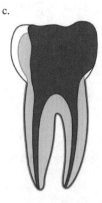

Figure 10.2

(a) Indication for indirect pulp cap-pulp not involved; (b) indication for pulpotomy-pulp inflamed or partially necrotic; (c) indication for pulpectomy-pulp completely necrotic.

（b 和 c 选自 *Dentistry at a Glance*, 1st Edition, Part 2, Chapter 60, Figures 60.3 and 60.4）

3.1　Indications

a. Co-operative child.

b. Compliant child and parent with regard to diet and oral hygiene.

c. Caries extending into the pulp in anaesthetised tooth.

d. No furcation involvement.

e. No abscess.

f. When extraction is not possible due to a bleeding disorder.

3.2　Contraindications

a. Tooth close to exfoliation.

b. Children who are immunosuppressed.

c. Children with congenital heart disease.

d. Poor general condition of the mouth, e.g., more than one or two teeth with likely pulpal involvement.

e. Insufficient coronal tooth tissue to ensure an effective coronal seal.

4. Devitalising Pulpotomy

This is a two-visit procedure used when adequate anaesthesia cannot be gained. At the first visit Ledermix paste on cotton wool is sealed into the cavity with a temporary cement for 7-14 days. At the second visit the necrotic pulp can be removed and restored as per a pulpectomy [3].

5. Pulpectomy

This is used when there is non-vital tissue in the root canals (Figure 10.2c). The canals are instrumented with files and then filled with zinc oxide cement or calcium hydroxide.

5.1 Indications

    a. Co-operative child.

    b. Compliant child and parent with regard to diet and oral hygiene.

    c. Irreversible pulpitis of primary molars.

    d. Pulp necrosis.

    e. Furcation involvement.

    f. Acute or chronic abscess.

    g. When a tooth needs to be maintained in the arch or extraction is contraindicated to due health reasons.

    h. No permanent successor.

5.2 Contraindications

    a. Medically compromised child.

    b. Poor general condition of the mouth, e.g., more than three teeth with likely pulpal involvement.

    c. Insufficient coronal tooth tissue to ensure an effective coronal seal.

    d. Tooth close to exfoliation.

Antibiotics may be administered, initially to relieve acute symptoms if there are systemic effects present or if there is an acute abscess or cellulitis present [4]. The pulpectomy can be performed following the subsidence of acute symptoms.

📄 Word List

1. radiograph [ˈreɪdɪəʊˌɡræf] *n.* 射线照片 *vt.* [核]拍射线照片
2. marginal ridge 边缘嵴
3. sinus [ˈsaɪnəs] *n.* 窦道
4. furcation [fəːˈkeɪʃən] *n.* 分歧；分支
5. radiolucency [ˌreɪdɪəʊˈljuːsənsɪ] *n.* 射线透射性；射线可透性
6. reversible pulpitis 可复性牙髓炎
7. irreversible pulpitis 不可复性牙髓炎
8. swelling [ˈswelɪŋ] *n.* 肿块；肿胀处
9. indirect pulp capping 间接盖髓术
10. vital pulpotomy 活髓切断术
11. desensitise [diːˈsensətaɪz] *v.* 使(病人或神经)对疼痛等无感觉或不敏感
12. lining [ˈlaɪnɪŋ] *n.* 衬层；内衬
13. secondary dentin 继发性牙本质
14. contraindication [ˌkɑːntrəˌɪndɪˈkeɪʃn] *n.* 禁忌证
15. linger [ˈlɪŋɡə(r)] *v.* 继续存留；缓慢消失；流连；逗留
16. anaesthetised [əˈnesθətaɪzd] *adj.* 被麻醉的
17. immunosuppressed [ˌɪmjunəʊsəˈprest] *adj.* 免疫抑制的
18. congenital heart disease 先天性心脏病
19. seal [siːl] *v.* 封上；密封 *n.* 印章；图章；密封物
20. Ledermix paste 一种由抗生素和类固醇构成的糊剂
21. cotton wool 药棉
22. pulp necrosis 牙髓坏死
23. root canal 根管
24. file [faɪl] *n.* 锉；锉刀
25. zinc oxide cement 氧化锌水门汀
26. calcium hydroxide 氢氧化钙
27. compliant [kəmˈplaɪənt] *adj.* 顺从的；服从的；符合的；一致的
28. oral hygiene 口腔卫生
29. medically compromised child 医疗条件受限的儿童
30. antibiotics [ˌæntɪbaɪˈɒtɪks] *n.* 抗生素

📝 Notes

❶ The aim of pulp therapy in deciduous teeth is to remove inflamed pulp tissue, conserve the damaged tooth and restore function until the permanent successor erupts.

乳牙牙髓治疗的目的是去除发炎的牙髓组织，保护受损的牙齿并恢复其功能，直到恒牙萌出。

❷ Irreversible pulpitis symptoms, e.g., pain waking child at night or pain that lingers without a stimulus.

不可逆牙髓炎的症状，例如儿童夜间痛，或无刺激因素导致的持续疼痛。

❸ At the first visit Ledermix paste on cotton wool is sealed into the cavity with a temporary cement for 7-14 days. At the second visit the necrotic pulp can be removed and restored as per a pulpectomy.

第一次就诊时，用暂封材料将带有 Ledermix 糊剂的棉球密封在髓腔中 7 至 14 天。第二次就诊时，可以按照牙髓切除术的方法去除坏死的牙髓并进行修复。

❹ Antibiotics may be administered, initially to relieve acute symptoms if there are systemic effects present or if there is an acute abscess or cellulitis present.

如存在全身症状，或出现急性脓肿或蜂窝组织炎，可先使用抗生素缓解急性症状。

（本单元由孟柳燕选编）

（文字部分选自 *Dentistry at a Glance*, 1st Edition, Part 2, Chapter 60）

Unit 11 ▸ Pulp Removal and Pulp Canal Obturation (Permanent Teeth)

1. Partial Pulp Removal (Pulpotomy)

Indications for partial pulp removal are:

a. Symptomatic irreversible pulpitis: partial pulp removal is as effective in relieving pain as pulpectomies. This is usually a temporary procedure, executed quickly in an emergency.

b. Incomplete root development: the aim of partial pulp removal is to amputate the coronal pulp in a tooth with incomplete root development while adding medication to encourage root growth and apical closure [1].

This technique has been used as a permanent procedure, applying a variety of medications to the root canal orifices followed by restoration. This is not universally approved of but deserves consideration when time, expertise and funds are available.

2. Complete Pulp Removal

Indications for complete pulp removal are:

a. Symptomatic irreversible pulpitis (pulpectomy).

b. Pulp necrosis (pulpal debridement).

3. Procedure for Pulp Removal

The availability of a pretreatment bitewing and at least one good periapical radiograph

本单元正文内容选自 Elizabeth Kay 所著 *Dentistry at a Glance*, John Wiley & Sons, Inc., 2016, Chapters 62 and 63, pp.130-133, 选用时 Chapter 63 有改动。

is essential before initiating pulp removal [2] (Figure 11.1a-c). The stages of pulp removal are:

　　a. Local anaesthesia.

　　b. Rubber dam isolation-this is mandatory.

　　c. Prepare occlusal access cavity for posterior teeth and lingual cavity for anterior teeth following the shape of the chamber and effectively removing its roof to allow straight-line access to the canal orifices (Figure 11.1d-f).

　　d. Debride pulp chamber and canals.

The length to which each canal should be cleaned and shaped (the working length) is determined either by taking radiographs with files in the canals and/or using electronic apex locators. Sufficient radiographs should be taken at different angles to determine the local anatomy in detail. The length should be measured from a reproducible reference point on the crown to the apical constriction (the cementodentinal junction). This point is not always discernible by tactile exploration but can be safely estimated as lying 0.5-1.5 mm from the radiographic root end (Figure 11.1g-1).

Shape and clean the canals as follows:

　　a. Widen the canal orifices and the coronal third of the canal (coronal flaring) by using hand or rotary instruments (Figure 11.2), allowing for minimal difficulty negotiating any curvature in the apical third.

　　b. There are many types of instruments available, both hand and rotary (Gates-Glidden drills, nickel-titanium files) (Figure 11.1m-o).

　　c. Confirm the working length as removing the curvature reduces the length of the canal.

　　d. Prepare the apical third of the canal to a size determined individually for each canal (Figure 11.2).

　　e. Prepare an apical 'stop' at or close to the cement-dentinal junction.

　　f. Shape the apical segment of the canal by either the 'crown down' or the 'step back' technique (Figure 11.2).

　　g. The apical constriction is likely to be absent in teeth with chronic periapical lesions as both bone and root resorption will have occurred. In such cases, an apical stop must be created artificially and is best placed further from the apex than it would be in a resorption-free root [3].

h. Recapitulate the filing to full working length between each step, including copious irrigation with sodium hypochlorite, using a file of the same size as the apical preparation (Figure 11.1p-r).

i. Rinse the canal with ethylene diamine tetracetic acid (17% EDTA) to remove dentinal debris.

j. If a second appointment is needed prior to obturation, the canals can be medicated with calcium hydroxide or antibiotic paste [4].

k. Place a cotton pellet in the pulp chamber and apply a sealing temporary restoration.

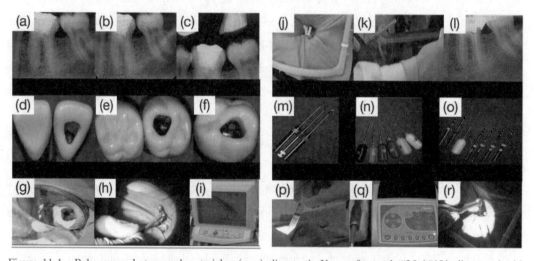

Figure 11.1　Pulp removal steps and materials: (a-c) diagnostic X-rays for tooth #36 (#19) diagnosed with necrosis and symptomatic apical periodontitis; (d) access opening on anterior tooth; (e) access opening on upper molar, buccal canal straight-line access; (f) palatal canal straight-line access; (g) access opening under rubber dam isolation, four canals found, distolingual canal access shown; (h,i) apex locator used to determine initial working length (WL); (j) four files placed, one for each canal; (k) distal angle X-ray taken to confirm WL; (l) working length X-ray, distal canals join and short; (m) Gates glidden drills for coronal flare; (n) hand file NiTi files (profile system); (o) protaper rotary NiTi system used for crown down technique, #15 file used to recapitulate; (p) copious irrigation with sodium hypochlorite used between files; (q) rotary file handpiece and control motor unit; (r) rotary instrumentation in progress.

(选自 *Dentistry at a Glance*, 1st Edition, Part 2, Chapter 62, Figure 62.1)

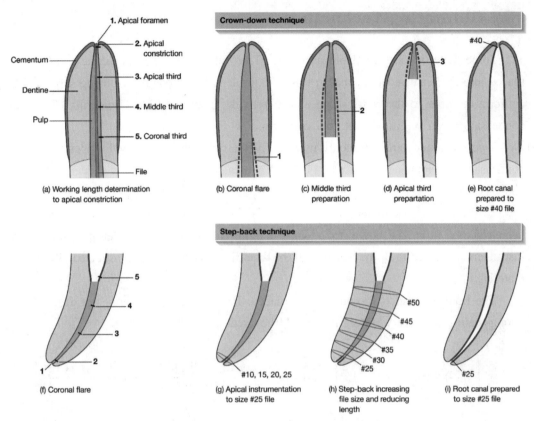

Figure 11.2 Pulpal removal/instrumentation techniques：（a）Working length determination to apical constriction. Crown-down technique；（b）Coronal flare；（c）Middle third preparation；（d）Apical third preparation；（e）Root canal prepared to #40 file. Step-Back technique：（f）Coronal flare；（g）Apical instrumentation to size #25 file；（h）Step-back increasing file size and reducing length；（i）Root canal prepared to size #25 file.

（选自 *Dentistry at a Glance*，1st Edition，Part 2，Chapter 62，Figure 62.2）

4. Aims of Pulp Obturation

Once the diseased pulp has been removed from a tooth and the pulp chamber and canal space cleaned and shaped these spaces should be obturated. The root canal obturation will impede the bacterial growth and favour the periapical healing.

5. Obturating Techniques

Some materials are available as cones. The initial cone (master cone) should be placed into the sealer-coated canal to full working length and condensed using spreaders to conform the cone to the canal shape and to provide space for further material [5]. This condensation can be carried out cold or warm.

Two techniques are commonly used to fill the remaining space with cones. In lateral condensation (Figures 11.3a-d and 11.4a, b), small cones are placed sequentially with condensation between each cone until the canal is filled. Excess cone is cut off at the canal orifices. In vertical condensation (Figures 11.3e-i and 11.4c-l), after the master cone has been placed, it is cut down to a short length and vertically condensed with warm instruments. The rest of the canal will be backfilled with thermoplasticised obturating material.

The final restoration should now be placed. If this is not possible or not desirable, a strong-sealing temporary restoration should be used.

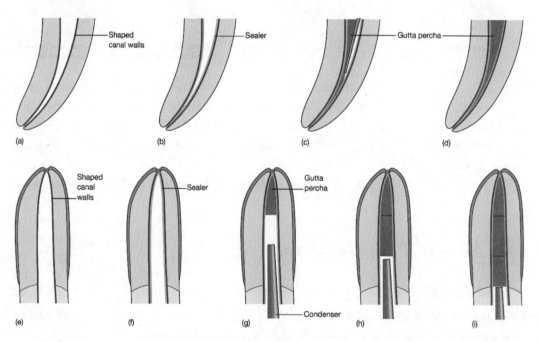

Figure 11.3　Obturating techniques

(a-d) Lateral condensation; (e-i) Vertical condensation. Red, shaped canal walls; yellow, sealer; pink, gutta percha; s, spreader; c, condenser.

(选自 *Dentistry at a Glance*, 1st Edition, Part 2, Chapter 63, Figure 63.1)

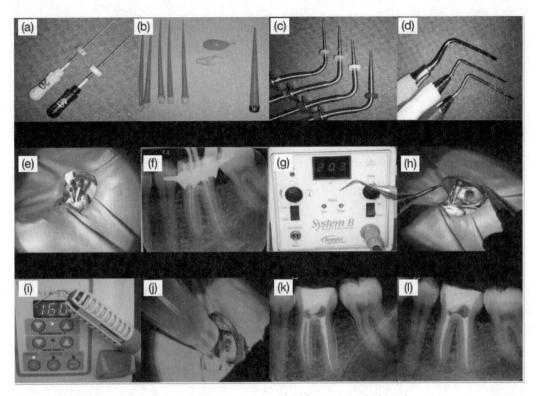

Figure 11.4   Instruments and materials for root canal obturation

（a）Finger spreaders for lateral condensation；（b）standardised gutta percha cones and cement；（c）heat spreader for vertical condensation；（d）condensers；（e）gutta percha master cones in place；（f）gutta percha master cones X-ray；（g）system B and heat spreader；（h）heat spreader inside the canal to remove part of the master cone；（i）thermoplastised gutta percha to back-fill the canal；（j）injection of themoplastised gutta percha in the canal；（k-l）final obturation X-rays.

（选自 *Dentistry at a Glance*, 1st Edition, Part 2, Chapter 63, Figure 63.2）

📄 Word List

1. execute［ˈeksɪkjuːt］ *v.* 执行；实施
2. amputate［ˈæmpjuteɪt］ *vt.* 切断
3. medication［ˌmedɪˈkeɪʃn］ *n.* 药物；药剂
4. root canal orifice 根管口
5. necrosis［neˈkrəʊsɪs］ *n.* 坏死
6. debridement［dɪˈbrɪdmənt］ *n.* 清创术；扩创术

7. anaesthesia [ˌænəsˈθiːzɪə] *n.* 麻醉

8. mandatory [ˈmændətərɪ] *adj.* 强制的；命令的

9. posterior teeth 后牙

10. anterior teeth 前牙

11. electronic apex locator 电子根尖定位仪

12. anatomy [əˈnætəmɪ] *n.* 解剖；解剖结构

13. cementodentinal junction 牙骨质界

14. discernible [dɪˈsɜːnəbl] *adj.* 可识别的；可辨别的

15. tactile [ˈtæktaɪl] *adj.* 触觉的；能触知的；有形的

16. curvature [ˈkɜːvətʃə(r)] *n.* 弯曲；弯曲部分

17. rinse [rɪns] *vt.* 漂洗；冲洗；漂净

18. ethylene diamine tetracetic acid 乙二胺四乙酸

19. debris [ˈdebriː] *n.* 残骸；碎屑

20. calcium hydroxide 氢氧化钙

21. antibiotic [ˌæntɪbaɪˈɒtɪk] *adj.* 抗生素的

22. paste [peɪst] *n.* 糊剂

23. apical periodontitis 根尖周炎

24. molar [ˈməʊlə(r)] *n.* 磨牙

25. buccal [ˈbʌkəl] *adj.* (面)颊的

26. palatal [ˈpælətl] *adj.* 腭的

27. distolingual [dɪstəʊˈlɪŋgwəl] *adj.* 远中舌的

28. coronal flare 冠状面

29. recapitulate [riːkəˈpɪtʃuleɪt] *v.* 重述；概括

30. copious [ˈkəʊpɪəs] *adj.* 大量的；丰富的

31. impede [ɪmˈpiːd] *vt.* 阻碍；妨碍；阻止

32. lateral condensation 侧方加压充填

33. vertical condensation 垂直加压充填

34. sealer [ˈsiːlə(r)] *n.* 封闭剂

35. gutta percha 牙胶

36. spreader [ˈspredə(r)] *n.* 侧压器

37. condenser [kənˈdensə(r)] *n.* 垂直加压器

38. cone [kəʊn] *n.* 圆锥形东西；圆锥体

39. backfill [ˈbækfɪl] *vt.* 回填

40. pulp chamber 髓腔；髓室

📝 Notes

❶ The aim of partial pulp removal is to amputate the coronal pulp in a tooth with incomplete root development while adding medication to encourage root growth and apical closure.

部分牙髓切断的目的是在牙根发育不全的患牙中切除冠髓，同时使用药物来促进牙根继续生长和根尖孔闭合。

❷ The availability of a pretreatment bitewing and at least one good periapical radiograph is essential before initiating pulp removal.

在开展牙髓摘除术前，必须有咬合翼片以及至少一张高质量的根尖片。

❸ In such cases, an apical stop must be created artificially and is best placed further from the apex than it would be in a resorption-free root.

在这样的病例中，必须人为地制作一个根尖止点，并且最好放置在比无牙根吸收区域的更远离根尖的位置。

❹ If a second appointment is needed prior to obturation, the canals can be medicated with calcium hydroxide or antibiotic paste.

如果需要在根管填充前进行第二次预约，可以用氢氧化钙或者抗生素糊剂对根管进行药物处理。

❺ The initial cone (master cone) should be placed into the sealer-coated canal to full working length and condensed using spreaders to confirm the cone to the canal shape and to prove space for further material.

应将初始牙胶尖(主牙胶尖)放入涂有封闭剂的根管中，直至整个工作长度，再使用侧方加压器加压主牙胶尖，确保牙胶尖与根管形态一致，并留出足够的空间容纳更多的材料。

(本单元由郭继华选编)

(文字部分选自 *Dentistry at a Glance*, 1st Edition, Part 2, Chapters 62 and 63)

Unit 12 Periodontium

12.1 The Normal Gingivae

The periodontium (Greek peri, around; odontos, tooth) comprises the tissues that support the teeth. The gingiva is the only one of the periodontal tissues that is visible. The major function of the gingiva is to provide a protective covering tissue, which maintains the integrity of the surface of the masticatory mucosa of the mouth. It is specialised to provide a junction with the tooth surface.

In health, the gingiva is pink with no swelling of the gingival margin (Figure 12.1A). Small depressions may be visible on the surface, giving it a stippled orange peel appearance. The gingival margin just covers the cement enamel junction (CEJ) of the teeth and runs parallel to it. The gingiva fills the spaces between the teeth, forming interdental papillae, which are limited by the contact points or contact areas between the neighbouring teeth. Melanin pigmentation may occur in response to local irritation from smoking (Figure 12.1B). The gingiva is continuous with the other mucosal tissues in the mouth. The mucogingival junction can be identified by the differences in colour and texture between the pink firm-textured gum tissue and the oral mucosa, which is red due to its rich, often visible network of underlying blood vessels, and has a looser texture (Figure 12.1A). The width of gum is measured from the gingival margin to the mucogingival junction (range 3-8 mm). Theoretically, a greater width helps to resist tension imposed on the gingival tissues by distension of the labial and buccal mucosae during eating. In the palate, the gingival tissues blend with the palatal mucosa. Local anatomical variations, such as frenal attachments, can intrude into the gingival tissue and

---

本单元正文内容选自 Elizabeth Kay 所著 *Dentistry at a Glance*, John Wiley & Sons, Inc., 2016, Chapters 34 and 35, pp.76-79。

reduce its width (Figure 12.1C). Variations in the gingival tissues, for example, how thick or thin they are, reflect genetic mechanisms responsible for the size and shape of the dental and oral tissues. In general, a thin gingival tissue biotype is more likely to be affected by gingival recession in response to traumatic stimulation from vigorous toothbrushing (Figures 12.1D and 12.1E).

Between the gingival tissue and the tooth, there is a shallow gingival sulcus, which can be measured by inserting a periodontal probe with gentle pressure, no greater than 30 g, which equates to the weight of the probe (Figure 12.1F). In the ideal situation, this sulcus is about 1 mm in depth; however, there is a normal range of variation, and it may be as deep as 3 mm. It should be appreciated that in most 'normal' cases we are examining clinically healthy gingival tissues, reflecting repeated exposure to dental plaque even in those with good oral hygiene.

The cellular structure of the gingiva is a key determinant of its protective function. It is made up of connective tissue covered with a stratified squamous epithelium (Figure 12.1G). The epithelial cells adhere to each other through specialised intracellular structures called desmosomes. One-half of the attachment (hemidesmosome) is contributed by each cell. Cells traverse the epithelium over a 1-month period after division in the basal layer. As the epithelial cells approach the surface, keratin forms in those cells, which are exposed to frictional forces from food during mastication. The cells in the basal layer of the epithelium are joined to the underlying connective tissue through a basement membrane. The epithelium can be differentiated into different compartments (oral, sulcular or junctional) depending on its position (see Figure 12.2A). The oral epithelium that covers the visible surface of the gum is keratinised. The gingival sulcus is lined by sulcular epithelium, which is not keratinised as it is not exposed to frictional forces. This blends with the junctional epithelium, which is attached via hemidesmosomes to the enamel down to the CEJ (Figure 12.1H).

The connective tissue supports the epithelium and contains a network of blood vessels, nerves and lymphatics [1]. Blood vessels provide nutrition but do not enter the epithelium. They carry circulating inflammatory cells such as polymorphonuclear leukocytes (PMNs) to the gingival tissue (Figure 12.1I and Figure 13.1D). Even in clinical health, small numbers of PMNs migrate through the tissues into the gingival crevice and so into the mouth. Lymphocytes in the connective tissue can change into plasma cells, which produce antibodies as a targeted response to bacterial antigens derived from dental plaque.

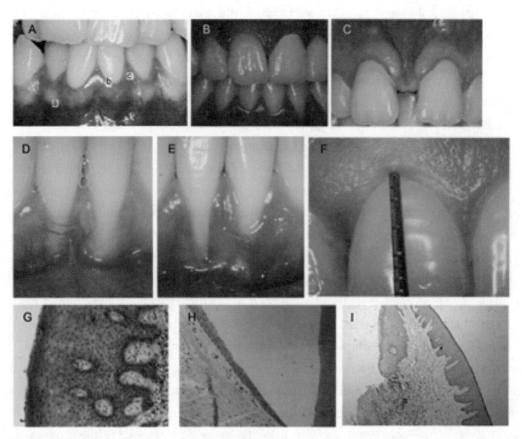

Figure 12.1　(A) Normal gingiva: a, the mucogingival junction identifies the border between the gingiva and the mucosa, which has a redder appearance and visible blood vessels; b, gingival margin; c, interdental papilla. (B) Gingival that has pigmentation related to a long-term smoking habit. (C) Gingival tissue with intrusive gingival frenum reducing the width of the gum. (D) Thin gingival tissues in a teenager; note the blood vessels visible through the thin labial gingival tissue of the lower right central incisor. (E) Gingival recession in the same patient 18 months later. (F) Probing a normal gingival sulcus; the sulcus is 1 mm deep measured with a conventional periodontal probe with Williams markings (1, 2, 3, 5, 7, 8, 9 mm); note no bleeding in response to gentle probing (G-H) histological sections of gum tissue: (G) oral epithelium with deeply stained surface parakeratinised layer; this is a stratified squamous keratinized epithelium on the external surface of the gingiva; (H) junctional epithelium 2-10 cells thick; the enamel has been removed during the preparation of the section leaving the underlying dentine. (I) Section of gingival tissue stained with haematoxylin and eosin: polymorphonuclear leukocytes, which have migrated from blood vessels into the connective tissue as a response to bacteria on the tooth surface (dental plaque), are present in large numbers as evidenced their darkly stained nuclei.

（选自 *Dentistry at a Glance*, 1st Edition, Part 2, Chapter 34, Figures 34.1-34.8）

Many of the mechanical properties of the gingiva depend on the structure of the connective tissue. Within a matrix of ground substance, the connective tissue contains fibroblasts, which are responsible for secreting collagen, the main structural protein. Collagen is organised into fibres, which are arranged in groups or bundles with a distinct orientation within the gingiva. The gingival connective tissue is attached to the surface of the alveolar bone and can be considered a mucoperiosteum.

The relationship between the tooth and the gingiva is unique as it represents the only part of the body in which a hard tissue is partly within the body (tooth root) and outside the body (tooth crown). There is a major challenge to ensure that there is no break in the integrity of the tissues, which would give bacteria direct access to the tissues with the possibility of recurrent infections. The integrity of the dentogingival junction is maintained by the junctional epithelium attachment to enamel (Figure 12.1I), further supported by the fibre structure in the connective tissue, which holds the gum tissue tightly against the tooth surface. It has been suggested that increased permeability of the junctional epithelium could increase the risk of bacterial toxins gaining access to the underlying connective tissue, leading to inflammation. However, this is only likely to be a factor when bacterial dental plaque has been allowed to accumulate over a period (see Figure 13.1C).

12.2 The Periodontal Ligament

The periodontal tissues include the gingiva, the periodontal ligament, the cementum covering the roots of the teeth, and the alveolar bone (Figure 12.2A). The major function of the periodontal tissues is to provide an attachment between the teeth and the bone of the jaws to facilitate mastication.

The surface of the roots is covered by a thin layer of cementum, which is a specialised mineralised tissue supported by the underlying dentine [2]. Cementum is made up of collagen fibres in an organic matrix and has a slightly higher mineral content (65%) than bone.

The alveolar bone exists to support the teeth and is maintained by the loading experienced during masticatory function. When teeth are extracted, the alveolar bone resorbs, leaving the basal bone of the jaws. In health, the alveolar bone does not extend to the cement enamel junction (CEJ), and the margin is located 1.5-2 mm below this landmark [3], leaving an extra-alveolar portion of the root.

The periodontal ligament (PDL) is a highly vascular connective tissue surrounding the roots of teeth, which joins the cementum to the alveolar bone of the socket wall [4].

The PDL contains sensory nerve fibres, lymphatics, and isolated epithelial cells (cell rests of Malassez), which are believed to be remnants of the embryonic root sheath. The width of PDL is 0.25 mm (range 0.2-0.4 mm). The collagen fibres of the PDL run into and become indistinguishable from the fibre structure of both cementum and alveolar bone (Figure 12.2B). The portions of the fibres within the mineralised tissues are called Sharpey fibres. The PDL contains fibre bundles named according to their orientation and position within the socket. The alveolar crest fibres run downwards and outwards from the extra-alveolar cementum to the bone margin; horizontal fibres run just below the alveolar crest; oblique fibres, which are the most numerous, run from cementum in an oblique direction to bone; and apical fibres radiate from cementum around the apex to bone. These fibre bundles allow forces from function or parafunction, tooth grinding or clenching, to be distributed to the alveolar bone.

Above the alveolar bone margin, the PDL is continuous with the connective tissue of the gingival tissues. In this extra-alveolar compartment, several groups of fibre bundles can be identified. The dentogingival fibres run from cementum into the connective tissue of the gingiva. There are, in addition: dentoperiosteal fibres (cementum to periosteum covering the alveolar bone); alveologingival fibres (alveolar bone into the gingival connective tissue); transeptal fibres (between the necks of neighbouring teeth above the alveolar crest); and circular fibres (encircle the teeth running in the gingival connective tissue). The main function of these extra-alveolar fibres is to strengthen the attachment of the gingiva to the tooth and the alveolar bone and therefore to provide support for the integrity of the dentogingival junction. In health, there are collagen fibres inserted into the cement covering the whole surface of the root (Figure 12.2C). In periodontitis, collagen fibres are lost below the CEJ, and the junctional epithelium migrates from enamel onto the root cementum (Figure 12.2D).

The walls of the sockets are cortical compact bone, and in radiographs, a radio-opaque line, termed the lamina dura, may be evident (Figure 12.2E). The external surface of the alveolar bone is also compact bone with the area between the socket wall and the surface occupied by cancellous spongy bone. The cancellous bone contains a high proportion of vascular connective tissue with bony struts termed trabeculae (Figure 12.2F). Blood vessels from cancellous bone run through canals (Volkmann's canals) in the socket wall into the PDL where they anastomose to provide a rich blood supply. The blood vessels are accompanied by sensory and proprioceptive nerve fibres. Proprioceptive mechanisms regulate chewing and protect the teeth from potential damage from sudden contact after biting through a hard component in food. The alveolar bone varies in

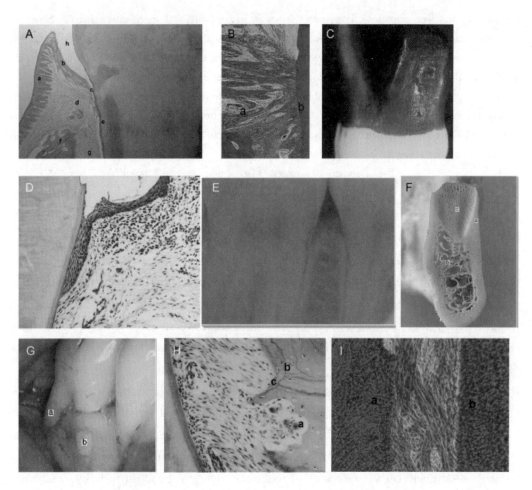

Figure 12. 2　（A）Histological section of a demineralised tooth showing periodontal tissues: a, oral epithelium; b, sulcular epithelium; c, junctional epithelium; d, gingival connective tissue; e, dentine covered by a thin layer of darkly stained cementum; f, alveolar bone which in health is located 1.5-2 mm below the cement-enamel junction; g, periodontal ligament; h, enamel space（enamel is a highly mineralised tissue with virtually no ground substance and so is not seen in histological sections which have been prepared by demineralising a tooth）.（B）Histological section showing: a, alveolar bone margin and b, root surface. The collagen fibres can be seen running into the cementum and the alveolar bone; the orientation of the fibre bundles is evident; Van Gieson stain for collagen.（C）Staining to show the collagen fibres which were broken when this carious tooth with a perfectly healthy periodontium was extracted; it is not possible to distinguish where the alveolar bone margin is on this tooth, showing that the collagen fibre attachment is the same in both the extra and intraalveloar portions of the root.（D）Periodontitis has resulted in loss of the attachment of fibres to the root cementum; the junctional epithelium has migrated on to the cementum and is now attached to it. Note also the presence of inflammatory cells, shown by the dark staining which represents their nuclei, in the connective tissue below the epithelium.（E）Radiograph showing a radio-opaque lamina dura outlining the compact bone forming the wall of the socket.（F）Section through the mandible showing

the socket of a lower premolar: a, compact bone of socket wall; b, cancellous trabecular bone; c, Volkmann's canals are visible in the socket wall. (G) Surgical flap raised to show lower first molar: a, prominent distal root with dehiscence of alveolar bone; b, fenestration (window) in alveolar bone over the mesial root (H-I) Tooth subjected to increased loading. (H) Resorption of alveolar bone by osteoclasts: a, the extent of the resorption can be visualised by darkly stained reversal lines in the bone, b, and it is on these surfaces that new bone is formed incorporating collagen fibres from the PDL, c. Haematoxylin and eosin staining. (I) Disordered arrangement of collagen fibres: fibres run into alveolar bone, a, and cementum, b. Van Gieson stain for collagen.

(选自 *Dentistry at a Glance*, 1st Edition, Part 2, Chapter 35, Figures 35.1-35.8)

thickness and is at its thinnest on the buccal of the upper canines and labial of the mandibular incisors. The alveolar bone margin may be deficient (termed a dehiscence) or there may be a window in the bone (termed a fenestration) (Figure 12.2G). Most often, this is genetically determined, resulting in a thin tissue biotype; however, it may be a result of a tooth root being displaced buccally, for example, in orthodontic treatment. The overall result is that increased areas of the roots are covered only by gingival tissues, which significantly increases the risk of gingival recession in response to stimuli such as vigorous toothbrushing.

The teeth are subjected to forces in normal function, and these are transmitted through the PDL to the alveolar bone. There is constant, rapid turnover in the PDL with breakdown and reformation of the collagen fibres, particularly those adjacent to the alveolar bone. There is also remodelling of the alveolar bone with resorption by specialised multinucleated giant cells (osteoclasts) balanced by new bone formed by osteoblasts (Figure 12.2H). The newly formed bone incorporates collagen fibres from the PDL and thus maintains the attachment to the socket wall. In parafunction, there is increased loading due to tooth-to-tooth contacts resulting from grinding and/or clenching. This results in changes in the PDL with an increased width of the ligament due to bone remodelling, particularly towards the alveolar bone margin, and increased turnover of the collagen with a resulting disordered orientation of the PDL fibres (Figure 12.2I). Clinically, there may be increased tooth mobility; however, there is no loss of collagen fibre attachment to the cementum of the root. The changes that take place in the tissues in response to increased loading are termed occlusal trauma. The remodelling of the alveolar bone in response to increased forces on the teeth is used to facilitate controlled tooth movement in orthodontics.

📋 Word List

1. gingiva [dʒɪnˈdʒaɪvə] *n.* 龈
2. cementum [sɪˈmentəm] *n.* 牙骨质
3. alveolar bone [ælˈviːələ bəʊn] *n.* 牙槽骨
4. calculus [ˈkælkjələs] *n.* 牙结石
5. epithelium [ˌepɪˈθiːlɪəm] *n.* 上皮
6. gingivitis [ˌdʒɪndʒɪˈvaɪtɪs] *n.* 龈炎
7. periodontitis [ˌperɪədɒnˈtaɪtɪs] *n.* 牙周炎
8. hemidesmosome [heˈmaɪdzmʊsəʊm] *n.* 半桥粒
9. collagen [ˈkɒlədʒən] *n.* 胶原蛋白
10. fibroblast [ˈfaɪbrəblæst] *n.* 成纤维细胞
11. mucoperiosteum [ˌmjuːkəʊperiˈɒstɪəm] *n.* 黏骨膜
12. desmosome [ˈdesməsəm] *n.* 桥粒
13. alveolar crest fibers [ælˈviːələ krest faɪbəz]. 牙槽嵴纤维
14. junctional epithelium [ˈdʒʌŋkʃənn(ə)l ˌepɪˈθiːlɪəm]. 结合上皮
15. periodontal probe [ˌperɪəˈdɒntl prəʊb]. 牙周探针
16. Sharpey fibers [ˈʃɑːpi faɪbəz] *n.* 夏比纤维
17. proprioceptive [prəʊprɪəˈseptɪv] *adj.* 本体感受的
18. periodontal pocket [ˌperɪəˈdɒntl ˈpɒkɪt]. 牙周袋

✍ Notes

❶ The connective tissue supports the epithelium and contains a network of blood vessels nerves and lymphatics.
结缔组织支撑上皮，并包含一个血管、神经和淋巴管网络。

❷ The surface of the roots is covered by a thin layer of cementum, which is a specialised mineralised tissue supported by the underlying dentine.
牙根表面覆盖着一层薄薄的牙骨质，这是由下层牙本质支撑的特殊矿化组织。

❸ In health, the alveolar bone does not extend to the cement enamel junction (CEJ) and the margin is located 1.5-2 mm below this landmark.

健康状态下，牙槽骨不延伸到牙骨质釉质交界处，边缘位于该标志以下 1.5~2 毫米处。

❹ The periodontal ligament（PDL）is a highly vascular connective tissue surrounding the roots of teeth which joins the cementum to the alveolar bone of the socket wall. 牙周韧带是一种高度血管化的结缔组织，包围牙根，将牙骨质与牙槽骨连接起来。

（本单元由刘欢选编）
（文字部分选自 *Dentistry at a Glance*，1st Edition，Part 2，Chapters 34 and 35）

Unit 13 ▸ Dental Plaque, Calculus and Diseases of the Gingivae and Periodontium

Dental plaque can be defined as a microbial community found on a tooth surface embedded in a matrix of polymers of bacterial and host origin (Figure 13.1A). It is a biofilm, which means it is a complex structure containing microorganisms that forms on surfaces immersed in an aqueous environment.

1. Plaque Formation

The tooth surface provides a unique non-shedding environment unlike the soft tissues in the oral cavity [1]. A clean tooth surface is rapidly covered by a layer of protein from saliva, termed the pellicle. Initial colonisation is by single bacterial cells, which have the ability to adhere to the pellicle. These primary colonisers are usually Gram-positive streptococci such as *Streptococcus sanguis*. These bacteria produce carbohydrate polymers, which they export to the extracellular environment as a matrix and acts as an energy store and provides anchoring material for further bacteria. Secondary colonisation occurs between 24 and 48 hours when species such as *Actinomyces naeslundii* attach to the primary colonisers (co-aggregation). In the absence of oral hygiene there is continued increase in the thickness of the plaque biofilm with division of bacteria to form colonies and further formation of extracellular matrix (Figure 13.1B). Poor diffusion of oxygen through the biofilm matrix means that it becomes anaerobic in its deeper layers. After a number of days an important step is colonisation by the *Fusobacterium nucleatum*, a key bridging bacterial species, which facilitates co-aggregation to incorporate late colonisers such as the Gram-negative anaerobe *Porphyromonas gingivalis*. Complexity thus increases and with time other Gram-negative anaerobic species can be incorporated into an established

本单元正文内容选自 Elizabeth Kay 所著 *Dentistry at a Glance*, John Wiley & Sons, Inc., 2016, Chapters 36 and 37, pp. 80-83。

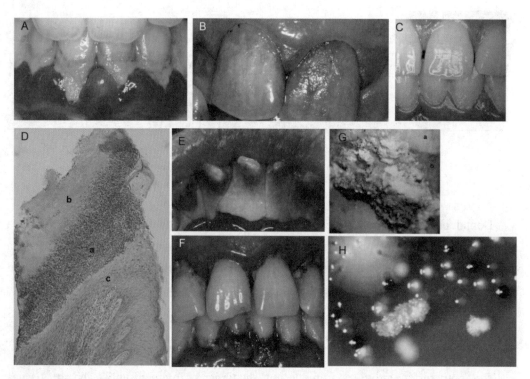

Figure 13.1 (A) Plaque present on the teeth in a patient with very poor oral hygiene; as the plaque gets thicker it becomes visible on examination. (B) Dental plaque biofilm after 3 days of undisturbed growth; clinically, the plaque would not be visible to the eye but can be seen after the application of a disclosing solution. (C) Undisturbed plaque accumulation related to the lower incisors for 14 days, in an experimental gingivitis model; there is associated swelling of the gingival margin resulting in the creation of a subgingival environment. Compare to gingival condition related to the upper teeth where there was normal plaque control. (D) Polymorphonuclear leukocytes (PMNs), which have migrated from blood vessels through the connective tissue into the gingival sulcus in response to bacterial plaque: a, a thick layer of PMNs visible by nuclear staining with haematoxylin; b, bacteria in dental plaque; c, gingival tissue. (E) Supragingival calculus related to the lingual surfaces of the lower incisor teeth. (F) Calculus, which was originally formed in a subgingival environment and is dark brown or black in colour; there is a layer of plaque on its surface. There has been gum recession in this patient as their periodontal disease has progressed, exposing the calculus. (G) Subgingival calculus, which is characteristically dark brown or black in colour and is below the cement enamel junction: a, enamel; b, root surface. It can be tenaciously attached to the root surface interlocking into small irregularities at the sites of former insertion of Sharpey's fibres, which have been exposed by the loss of periodontal attachment fibres. (H) Culture of bacteria from a periodontal pocket on blood agar showing black pigmented colonies of *Porphyromonas gingivalis*; this and other species that can produce pigment are responsible for the dark brown or black colour of subgingival calculus.

（选自 *Dentistry at a Glance*，1st Edition，Part 2，Chapter 36，Figures 36.1-36.8）

stable biofilm. Undisturbed plaque accumulation for 14 days, in an individual with initially healthy gingival tissue, will result in inflammation and provides a model of experimental gingivitis (Figure 13.1C).

Tissue changes, which occur as periodontal disease progresses, provide environmental niches that encourage the development of complex biofilms. A subgingival environment such as a periodontal pocket is protected from frictional forces associated with mastication and is inaccessible to plaque control. There will be differences in nutrition, with increased availability of blood serum via the gingival crevicular fluid (GCF) and reduced levels of oxygen. Motile bacteria, such as the spirochaete *Treponema denticola*, will be found in the GCF within a pocket. This organism can co-aggregate with other Gram-negative anaerobes in mature plaque. Biofilms represent the preferred method of growth for bacteria. Advantages include protection from competing microorganisms and from host defence mechanisms such as the influx of polymorphonuclear leukocytes (PMN) (Figure 13.1D). Mature intact biofilms are resistant to the effects of antibiotics and antiseptics, which cannot penetrate them to kill bacteria, and the cornerstone of treatment is mechanical disruption.

Calculus can be defined as mineralised bacterial plaque. It forms when bacteria in the deepest layers of plaque die and their cell bodies become mineralised by various crystalline forms of calcium phosphate. Supragingival calculus is creamy whitish to dark yellow in colour and is chalky in consistency (Figure 13.1E). It forms in plaque exposed to salivary secretions adjacent to the ducts of salivary glands and is particularly found on the lingual surface of lower incisors. Subgingival calculus is brownish black and provides an ideal surface for bacterial adhesion and further plaque growth (Figure 13.1G). Calculus acts as a plaque-retentive factor and subgingival calculus in particular keeps the plaque biofilm in close contact with the soft tissue surface of the wall of the periodontal pocket (Figure 13.1F).

2. Specific Bacterial Species and Periodontitis

About 700 different bacterial species can be identified in the oral cavity and many are commensal bacteria, which exist in harmony with the host [2]. Investigations of mature subgingival plaque biofilms have identified specific groupings of bacterial species. The 'red complex', which consists of *Porphyromonas gingivalis*, *Tannerella forsythia* and

Treponema denticola, have been found to be strongly associated with each other (co-aggregation) and with diseased sites (Figure 13.1H). *Porphyromonas gingivalis* is strongly associated with periodontal disease but is not a potent inducer of inflammation. Experimental studies suggest it is a keystone microorganism, which even in very low numbers can subvert the host response leading to a major increase in commensal microbial load, resulting in periodontal destruction. *Porphyromonas gingivalis* is also present in bacterial biofilms that are not associated with disease. It is possible that pathogenicity may depend on the specific strain of the bacteria; alternatively, the host response may be able to attenuate the capacity of bacteria to cause disease.

Localised aggressive periodontitis (LAP) is a rare type of periodontal disease (see Figure 13.2I). The bacterial species *Aggregatibacter actinomycetemcomitans* is almost always recovered from samples taken from affected individuals. A specific clone of this bacteria, the JP2 clone, was identified in populations from Mediterranean Africa. This clone has a genetic mutation and it produces very high levels of leukotoxin, which substantially suppresses PMN function. A prospective 2-year study of teenage schoolchildren in Morocco found that carriers of the JP2 clone of *Aggregatibacter actinomycetemcomitans* at baseline were 18 times more likely to develop LAP and 70% of those with JP2 developed this condition. The study was the first clear demonstration that a specific bacterial species caused periodontal disease, albeit a rare form of the condition.

3. Diseases of the Gingivae and Periodontium

Diseases of the periodontal tissues are among the most common to affect mankind. Gingivitis, a chronic inflammatory condition, represents the response of the gingiva to the accumulation of dental plaque on the surface of the teeth. Those affected will often complain of bleeding gums, particularly in response to toothbrushing or after eating, but the condition is not usually painful (see Figure 13.1C). Gingivitis is a reversible condition and the removal of dental plaque and calculus will result in a return to gingival health [3]. Gingival inflammation is very common and is evident to some degree in virtually all adolescents at puberty, followed by a reduction in its prevalence. It is not the case that all individuals with poor plaque control and persistent gingivitis will progress to periodontitis. Inflammatory changes may be present for many years with limited or no involvement beyond the gingival tissues (contained gingivitis), which fits with the concept that inflammation is a protective response (Figure 13.2A). Hormonal influences mean that there is increased expression of gingivitis during pregnancy. There may be localised inflammatory swellings (pregnancy epulis), which regress after childbirth (Figure 13.2B). In other cases, a definitive diagnosis for a localised swelling of the gingival margin will require a histopathological examination of the excised tissue. Fibrous epulis is the most common diagnosis for such swellings.

Chronic periodontitis can be defined as loss of support of the affected teeth due to loss of connective tissue attachment and alveolar bone [4]. It results in irreversible destruction of components of the periodontal tissues that support the teeth. Chronic periodontitis is not usually painful and often does not become evident to affected individuals until they notice loosening, or a change in the position, of one or more of their teeth. There is considerable variation between different populations with 5%-20% of adults suffering from periodontal disease at a level that requires some treatment. As periodontitis develops, there are changes in the tissues, which mean that periodontal pockets become deeper and this forms the basis for the basic periodontal examination (BPE) that is used as a screening method to identify periodontal disease and the specific treatment required (Figures 13.2C and 13.2D). Deepened periodontal pockets provide the ecological niche to support the incorporation of anaerobic Gram-negative microorganisms into the subgingival dental plaque biofilm, increasing the likelihood of progressive periodontal disease. However, ultimately it is loss of periodontal attachment, measured from the cement enamel junction to the bottom of the pocket, which provides a measure of the severity of periodontitis. Chronic periodontitis is often associated with poor oral hygiene, generalised plaque, calculus and obvious inflammatory changes in the gingival tissues (Figure 13.2E). Localised infection within a deep periodontal pocket can result in the formation of a periodontal abscess (Figure 13.2F). Drainage of pus can usually be established through the pocket. A careful examination is indicated to distinguish this from a periapical abscess.

The absence of obvious signs of inflammation of the gingival margin cannot be used to exclude periodontitis [5]. As periodontitis progresses, the inflammatory component is located subgingivally at the bottom of the periodontal pocket and there may be no sign of changes affecting the gingival margin. It is therefore important to examine the periodontal tissues in adults using a screening system, such as the BPE, to exclude periodontitis. There are risk factors that are associated with increased prevalence and severity of periodontitis, in particular smoking, which has been implicated in more than 50% of all cases of periodontitis. Smoking suppresses the inflammatory response allowing periodontitis to progress particularly on surfaces where there is direct contact with cigarette smoke. Thus the pattern of periodontal destruction in smokers often includes the anterior teeth and in particular the palatal surfaces of the upper teeth (Figure 13.2G).

Aggressive periodontitis is a rare condition representing periodontitis that progresses rapidly and occurs in young individuals. Although uncommon, it has considerable significance as it often affects the very young and may result in tooth loss. Localised aggressive periodontitis is most often reported in adolescents where extensive periodontal destruction typically affects a small number of teeth, including the first molars and incisors (Figure 13.2I). Generalised aggressive periodontitis tends to be identified in those aged below 35 years and affects many of the teeth (Figure 13.2J). It is generally accepted that there is a strong genetic link in aggressive periodontitis, probably having an effect by suppressing appropriate inflammatory or immune responses to causative bacteria. Alternatively, specific virulent bacteria may suppress the host response. Genetic factors may explain the variations worldwide, with a high prevalence in populations from parts of Africa and a very low prevalence in Caucasians.

Acute ulcerative gingivitis (AUG) is a condition that affects young individuals and presents with pain, tenderness, spontaneous gingival bleeding and complaints of halitosis. It often affects the lower incisor region and the loss of gingival contour due to necrosis of interdental papillae is a distinctive feature (Figure 13.2H). Smoking is present in virtually all cases and is associated with other risk factors, including poor oral hygiene and stress. There is a specific anaerobic flora in AUG with fusobacteria and spirochaetes. AUG responds rapidly to antibiotics, particularly metronidazole, followed by periodontal treatment; however, rapid recurrence is common if the risk factors persist. Occasionally, if AUG does not respond to treatment, it is associated with systemic diseases that impair immunity such as HIV.

Leukaemias represent the malignant proliferation of white blood cells and can be acute or chronic. These can present as gingival swelling, due to the accumulation of white blood cells in the gingival tissues, or excessive and persistent bleeding, due to secondary thrombocytopenia (decreased platelets) (Figure 13.2K). A rapid diagnosis is important and blood tests will identify whether a leukaemia is present.

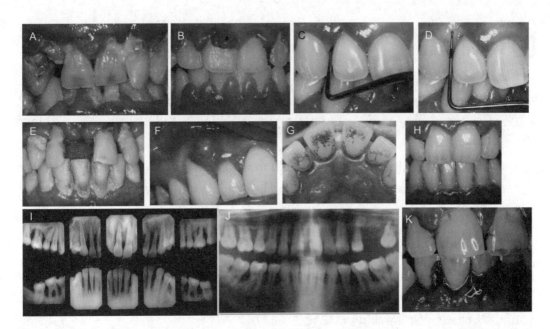

Figure 13.2   (A) Contained gingivitis: this 72-year-old man presented with pain from a carious upper incisor. He never brushed his teeth as he was too busy with his job running a farming business. He had very obvious gingivitis but little evidence of involvement of the periodontal tissues with loss of periodontal attachment. (B) Gingivitis in a 22-year-old who was in the third month of her pregnancy. It represents an exaggerated response to dental plaque, which is visible on the teeth: a, localised swelling of the gingival margin related to the upper right central incisor, which is termed a pregnancy epulis. (C-D) Assessment of the periodontal status using the basic periodontal examination: (C) World Health Organisation (WHO) probe in a periodontal pocket; (D) there is bleeding after the probe has been removed showing active inflammation. The band on the probe is between 3.5 and 5.5 mm from the ballended tip. (E) Chronic periodontitis in a 45-year-old man with very poor oral hygiene and gross plaque accumulation. (F) A fluctuant swelling of the buccal gingiva in a 50-year-old female related to a periodontal abscess; this represents an infection in a deep pocket on the mesiobuccal surface of the upper right canine. An abscess is defined as a circumscribed collection of pus. (G) This 43-year-old woman was complaining of spacing, which had developed between her upper incisors over the preceding year. She had a good standard of plaque control and no evidence of gingival inflammation. Subgingival calculus deposits are evident on the palatal surfaces of the incisors and there was deep pocketing. The woman had smoked 20 cigarettes per day for over 20 years. Note also the glazed appearance of the palatal tissues. (H) Acute ulcerative gingivitis in an 18-year-old female who smoked 15 cigarettes per day. She was complaining of pain in her gums and marked halitosis. Note the loss of the interdental papillae, which is a characteristic presentation of this condition. (I) Radiograph showing vertical bone loss affecting the first molar and incisor teeth in a 15-year-old boy; the diagnosis was advanced localised aggressive periodontitis. (J) Radiographic appearance of a 28-year-old woman with generalized aggressive periodontitis. She presented because a space had developed between her upper central incisors over a 9-month period. Note the generalised advanced bone loss. (K) Acute myeloid leukaemia in a 45-year-old man who had been complaining of blood oozing from his gums for a month. He had attended his doctor on two occasions before being referred for a dental opinion. A blood test identified the need for onward referral for specialist management but despite chemotherapy, he died 2 months later.

（选自 *Dentistry at a Glance*, 1st Edition, Part 2, Chapter 37, Figures 37.1-37.9）

📄 Word List

1. gingival crevicular fluid（GCF）［dʒɪnˈdʒaɪvəl ˈkrevɪkjʊlə ˈfluːɪd］龈沟液

2. polymorphonuclear leukocytes（PMN）［ˌpɒliˌmɔːfəˈnjuːkljə ˈljuːkəsaɪt］多形核白细胞

3. fusobacterium nucleatum［ˌfjuːzəʊbækˈtɪəriəm ˌnjuːkliˈætəm］核梭杆菌

4. porphyromonas gingivalis［ˌpɔːfɪrəˈməʊnəs ˌdʒɪndʒɪˈvælɪs］牙龈卟啉单胞菌

5. tannerella forsythia［ˌtænəˈrɛlə fɔːˈsaɪθɪə］福赛氏坦纳菌

6. treponema denticola［ˌtrɛpəˈniːmə ˌdɛntɪˈkoʊlə］齿垢螺旋体

7. biofilm［ˈbaɪəʊfɪlm］n. 生物膜

8. actinomyces naeslundii［ˌæktɪˈnəʊmaɪsiːz ˌnɛsˈlʌndɪˌaɪ］奈瑟氏放线菌

9. pellicle［ˈpelɪkl］n. 薄膜

10. spirochaete［ˈspaɪərəkiːt］n. 螺旋体

11. aggregatibacter actinomycetemcomitans［ˌægrɪɡeɪtəˈbæktə(r) ˌæktɪˌnəʊmaɪˈsɛtəm ˌkɒmɪˈtænz］集聚放线菌

12. leukotoxin［ˌljuːkəʊˈtɒksɪn］n. 白细胞毒素

13. commensal bacteria［kəˈmensl bækˈtɪərɪə］共生细菌

14. keystone microorganism［ˈkiːstoʊn ˌmaɪkroʊˈɔːɡənɪzəm］基石微生物

15. subgingival［ˌsʌbdʒɪnˈdʒaɪrəl］adj. 龈下的

16. periodontal abscess［ˌperiəˈdɒntl ˈæbses］牙周脓肿

17. periapical abscess［pɪəˈraɪəpɪkl ˈæbses］根尖脓肿

18. occlusal trauma［əˈkluːs(ə)l ˈtrɔːmə］咬合创伤

19. tooth mobility［tuːθ məʊˈbɪləti］牙齿松动

20. probing depth［ˈprəʊbɪŋ depθ］探诊深度

21. gingival margin［dʒɪnˈdʒaɪvəl ˈmaːdʒɪn］龈缘

22. periodontal charting［ˌperiəˈdɒntl ˈtʃaːtɪŋ］牙周记录

23. periodontal dressing［ˌperiəˈdɒntl ˈdresɪŋ］牙周敷料

24. furcation involvement［fɜːˈkeɪʃən ɪnˈvɒlvmənt］分叉病变

25. scaling and root planing［ˈskeɪlɪŋ ənd ruːt ˈpleɪnɪŋ］刮治和根面平整

26. guided tissue regeneration［ˈɡaɪdɪd ˈtɪʃuː riˈdʒenəreɪʃən］引导组织再生

27. periodontal maintenance［ˌperiəˈdɒntl ˈmeɪntənəns］牙周维护

28. gingival graft［dʒɪnˈdʒaɪvəl graːft］牙龈移植

29. osseous surgery［ˈɒsɪəs ˈsɜːdʒəri］骨手术

30. plaque control [plæk kənˈtroul] 牙菌斑控制
31. dental calculus removal [ˈdentl ˈkælkjələs rɪˈmuːvl] 牙结石去除
32. interdental papilla [ˌɪntə(ː)ˈdentl pəˈpɪlə] 龈乳头
33. gingival fibers [dʒɪnˈdʒaɪvəl ˈfaɪbəz] 牙龈纤维

📝 Notes

❶ The tooth surface provides a unique non-shedding environment unlike the soft tissues in the oral cavity.
牙齿表面提供了一个独特的不脱落环境，不同于口腔中的软组织。

❷ About 700 different bacterial species can be identified in the oral cavity and many are commensal bacteria which exist in harmony with the host.
口腔中可以识别出约 700 种不同的细菌，许多是与宿主和谐共存的共生细菌。

❸ Gingivitis is a reversible condition and the removal of dental plaque and calculus will result in a return to gingival health.
龈炎是一种可逆的状态，去除牙菌斑和牙结石将恢复牙龈健康。

❹ Chronic periodontitis can be defined as loss of support of the affected teeth due to loss of connective tissue attachment and alveolar bone.
慢性牙周炎可以定义为由于结缔组织附着和牙槽骨的丧失导致患牙失去支撑。

❺ The absence of obvious signs of inflammation of the gingival margin cannot be used to exclude periodontitis.
牙龈缘没有明显的炎症迹象不能用来排除牙周炎。

(本单元由曹正国选编)

(文字部分选自 *Dentistry at a Glance*, 1st Edition, Part 2, Chapters 36 and 37)

Unit 14 ▶ Caries Prevention and Plaque Reduction

1. Caries Prevention

Caries is the localized destruction of susceptible dental hard tissues by acidic by-products from the bacterial fermentation of dietary carbohydrates. It is one of the most common diseases worldwide and people remain susceptible throughout life.

Despite significant improvements in oral health in the UK over the past 30 years, the burden of caries remains unacceptably high in many communities and has wide social and economic consequences. Dental professionals have an important role in delivering prevention in the clinical setting for individual patients. However, effectively preventing caries in the population requires policies that address all risk factors at all levels of society.

The caries process is multifactorial and dynamic and it is possible to arrest or reverse early lesions before cavitation occurs [1]. The contemporary view of the caries process is that it is controllable, and as such all patients should receive preventive advice and treatment. Caries risk assessment, where a patient is assigned to a risk category (usually high or low) is an essential element of caries control.

1.1 Caries Control

Figure 14.1 shows the biology of caries. There are two broad approaches to caries control: (1) strengthening or protecting the tooth and (2) behavior modification to reduce the availability of substrate and promote the regular removal of plaque [2]. In practice, caries control is achieved through the following actions.

本单元正文内容选自 Elizabeth Kay 所著 *Dentistry at a Glance*, John Wiley & Sons, Inc., 2016, Chapters 22 and 23, pp.48-51. 选用时图表有删除,文字有少量变动。

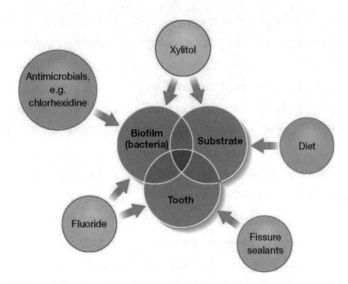

Figure 14.1 Biology of caries

（选自 *Dentistry at a Glance*, 1st Edition, Part 2, Chapter 22, Figure 22.1）

1.1.1 Plaque Control

Regular disturbance of the biofilm by toothbrushing prevents plaque accumulation and is the principal vehicle for introducing fluoride to teeth [3]. Brushing twice per day is a social norm for the majority of people. For some patients, physical plaque removal is problematic and it may be supplemented by the use of the antimicrobial chlorhexidine. While regular professional prophylaxis has been shown to be effective, it is neither a practical nor cost-effective caries control measure.

1.1.2 Diet

The aim of dietary advice is to reduce the amount of sugar consumed and the frequency of its intake. Free sugars found in food and drinks are the most important dietary factors. Standard advice is to restrict their intake to mealtimes only (three to four times a day) and not within 1 hour of going to bed. For dietary advice to be effective it must be personal, concise, and positive and a 3-day diet diary is a method of working with patients to modify their diet. Dietary advice should also include information on healthy nutrition and should always be given in the wider context of general health.

1.1.3 Fluoride

Fluoride has been proven effective in caries prevention. It has a systemic and topical anticaries effect, providing the greatest protection to the smooth surfaces of teeth when present topically in the mouth at frequent low doses. It has several anticaries properties but the principal action when present in plaque fluid is to promote remineralization over demineralization in the caries process [4]. The effectiveness of fluoride is dose (concentration) dependent, with higher concentrations offering greater caries reductions. However, this must be balanced against its associated risks. Swallowing and eating toothpaste during dental development can lead to mottling (fluorosis), which in severe cases can be unaesthetic. Acute overdose can also occur if fluoride ingestion is excessive, leading to systemic toxicity at doses of 1 mg/kg or even death if doses exceed 5 mg/kg[5]. For this reason, prescribing fluoride should be based on caries risk and existing exposure. National guidelines are available to assist in this process.

1.1.4   Sealants

Fissure sealants can be applied to the non-cleaning pit and fissure surfaces of susceptible teeth. For maximum benefit, they should be applied as soon as possible after eruption. There is a good evidence that sealing permanent molar teeth in children and adolescents at high risk of caries is an effective preventive measure. However, placement of fissure sealants is technique sensitive, and even when successfully applied they require careful monitoring and repair to ensure the all-important seal is maintained.

1.1.5   Xylitol

Xylitol is an artificial sweetener commonly used as a replacement for sugar. Xylitol is non-acidogenic and has anticaries properties due to antimicrobial actions [6]. When contained in gum, the action of chewing also stimulates saliva flow for additional caries protection. Chewing sugar-free gum after meals is therefore recommended for at-risk patients. Its use, however, should be avoided in young children and can produce side effects if used to excess in other age groups.

1.1.6   The Dental Team

The adoption of a preventive philosophy is fundamental to caries control. Important factors include the use of skill mix (the wider dental team) to support patients in adopting new behaviors and habits, early diagnosis of caries using radiographs as appropriate, and conservative management of early lesions in an attempt to prevent their progression to cavitation. It is important to implement relevant prevention strategies based on the best available evidence. Clinical guidelines aid treatment planning based on an individual's caries risk assessment. The interval for dental recall should also be linked to a patient's risk status, so those at high risk of caries are recalled more frequently for examination and preventive care [7].

1.1.7   The Public Health Approach

Clinical practice is only partially successful in caries prevention because individual behaviors are shaped by social and environmental factors—the social determinants of health. Professional actions are also only relevant to those people regularly accessing dental care. For this reason, partnership working and the use of multidisciplinary teams are vital to engaging communities to reduce risk factors for caries [8]. This involves working with other health professionals, such as health visitors and school nurses, and alongside other programs to ensure activities to reduce caries are integral to general health improvement activities. Outreach working has grown in recent years whereby dental professionals support or deliver interventions in the community setting. Programs may include fluoride in their design via supervised toothbrushing clubs or the professional application of fluoride varnish to the teeth of children in nurseries and schools.

2. Plaque Reduction

2.1 Mechanical

2.1.1　The Public Health Approach

Manual toothbrushing is currently the most commonly used oral hygiene measure. Twice daily toothbrushing for 2 minutes should be performed to ensure the removal of plaque. A medium-filament small flat-headed brush is recommended and some authorities recommend changing the toothbrush every 3 months, although there is no evidence that this is critical to plaque removal [9]. Modifications to the shape of the head, including concave heads and double and triple-headed brushes, have also been proposed. Double and triple-headed toothbrushes have been shown to be more effective in the removal of plaque on lingual surfaces but these are not widely used.

A number of toothbrushing techniques have been described but there is no good evidence for one technique over another. Where a patient's toothbrushing technique requires modification, the modified Bass technique has been found to be effective. This involves brushing with the bristles angled at 45° to the tooth with a small circular or vibrating motion. This systematic approach ensures that all areas of the mouth are covered. In clinical studies, toothbrushing alone has been shown to remove between 39% and 50% of plaque and to result in a 35% reduction in gingival bleeding [10].

Powered toothbrushes that work in an oscillating, rotating fashion have been recently shown to have improved efficacy when compared with manual toothbrushes. Brushes using sonic technology are also available and are also effective at removing plaque. These brushes utilize acoustic vibrations and dynamic fluid activity to remove plaque. Patients with limited manual dexterity, those caring for mentally handicapped patients, or orthodontic patients could consider a powered brush. Powered brushes have also been shown to enhance long-term compliance and so might be suitable for patients who are unable to achieve good plaque control using a manual brush [11]. The cost of high-end powered toothbrushes needs to be balanced against the perceived clinical benefit.

2.1.2　Interdental Cleaning

Effective toothbrushing can only clean around 65% of the tooth surface as it only removes plaque from the buccal, lingual, and occlusal surfaces. Periodontitis occurs primarily between teeth; therefore, interdental cleaning is always necessary. Interdental cleaning can be performed using dental floss, dental tape, interdental brushes, toothpicks, or powered irrigation devices. Studies have shown that the addition of interdental cleaning reduces bleeding on probing by 67% compared with 35% using toothbrushing alone. Interdental plaque should be removed at 12 to 48-hour intervals so daily interdental cleaning is therefore recommended [12].

Flossing can be carried out using either waxed floss or tape and there is no evidence to suggest either is more efficient at plaque removal. Floss is best used in sites where there has been little or no interdental recession and where the papilla fills the interdental space. Triangular toothpicks or wood sticks with a low surface hardness and high strength have been shown to be most effective where there is some recession.

Where space permits, interdental brushes are preferred, as they are more effective at cleaning grooves on exposed root surfaces. Interdental brushes can remove plaque up to 2.5 mm below the gingival margin and can clean areas that would be inaccessible to floss once the recession has occurred. In addition, patients are more likely to comply with interdental brush use than floss. Interdental brushes come in a variety of sizes and advice from a dental professional will help the patient choose the correct brush size. Interdental cleaning aids should be reviewed as treatment progresses because the resolution of inflammation will lead to recession and an increase in the size of interdental embrasure spaces.

2.2　Chemical Plaque Reduction

Levels of dental plaque can also be reduced by chemical antiplaque agents. While these can be administered through a variety of vehicles, toothpaste and mouth rinses are the most commonly used. The efficacy of antiplaque agents is not directly related to antimicrobial action but rather seems to be related to persistence of action or substantivity.

2.2.1　Chlorhexidine Gluconate

Chlorhexidine was the earliest and one of the most effective antiplaque agents available. It is a dicationic bisbiguanide available in 0.12% and 0.2% preparations for twice daily use [13]. Adverse effects reported include staining of teeth, mucositis, reversible epithelial desquamation, alteration of taste, salivary gland swelling, and increased supragingival calculus.

2.2.2　Quaternary Ammonium Compounds

Cetylpyridinium chloride (0.05%) is the most studied of the quaternary ammonium compounds. The duration of action is only 3-5 hours and, although some plaque inhibitory effect has been shown, most studies have concluded that it has a minimal effect on gingivitis when used in conjunction with toothbrushing. Cetylpyridinium chloride is also associated with staining of the teeth with regular use.

2.2.3　Phenolic Compounds and Essential Oils

Triclosan: This is a non-ionic antimicrobial. It is found mainly in toothpastes and mouthrinses at 0.2%-0.3% and has a substantivity of 5 hours. The activity of triclosan is increased by the addition of zinc citrate or polyvinyl methyl ethyl maleic acid (PVM/MA). Long-term reduction in plaque averaged between 20% and 40% and in gingivitis 20%-40%. Some studies have shown that triclosan and co-polymer have an anti-inflammatory effect that is independent of their antimicrobial effect. Studies have shown a modest beneficial effect on the progression of periodontitis.

Essential Oils: Combinations of essential oils have been shown to be effective chemical adjuncts to plaque control. Strong taste, a low pH, a burning sensation in the mucosa, and a high alcohol concentration are reported.

2.2.4　Stannous Fluoride

Stannous fluoride has been shown to reduce gingival inflammation and bleeding, although it has less of an effect on plaque levels. It is possible that it exerts its anti-inflammatory effect through modifying the plaque rather than removing it [14]. Other antiplaque and gingivitis agents that have been evaluated include metal salts, oxygenating agents, detergents, amine alcohols (delmopinol), salifluor, acidified sodium chlorite, and hexetidine.

📄 Word List

1. acidic [əˈsɪdɪk] *adj.* 酸性的
2. multifactorial [ˌmʌltɪfækˈtɔːrɪəl] *adj.* 多因素的
3. dynamic [daɪˈnæmɪk] *adj.* 动态的；发展变化的
4. controllable [kənˈtrəʊləbl] *adj.* 可控制的
5. prophylaxis [ˌprɒfəˈlæksɪs] *n.* 预防性清洁术
6. topical [ˈtɒpɪkl] *adj.* 局部的
7. dental fluorosis 氟牙症
8. unaesthetic [ˌʌniːsˈθetɪk] *adj.* 无美感的
9. eruption [ɪˈrʌpʃ(ə)n] *n.* 萌出
10. sealant [ˈsiːlənt] *n.* 封闭剂
11. xylitol [ˈzaɪlɪtɒl] *n.* 木糖醇
12. acidogenic [ˌæsɪdəʊˈdʒenɪk] *adj.* 产酸的
13. individual's caries risk assessment 个性化龋病风险评估
14. multidisciplinary [ˌmʌltɪdɪsəˈplɪnərɪ] *adj.* 多学科的
15. concave [kɒnˈkeɪv] *adj.* 凹面的
16. gingival bleeding 牙龈出血
17. powered toothbrushes 电动牙刷
18. manual toothbrushes 手动牙刷
19. oscillating [ˌɒsɪˈleɪtɪŋ] *adj.* 振荡的
20. rotating [rəʊˈteɪtɪŋ] *adj.* 旋转的
21. sonic [ˈsɒnɪk] *adj.* 声波的
22. acoustic [əˈkuːstɪk] *adj.* 声音的
23. vibration [vaɪˈbreɪʃn] *n.* 震动；颤动
24. dynamic fluid 动态流体
25. dexterity [dekˈsterətɪ] *n.* 灵巧；敏捷
26. handicapped [ˈhændɪkæpt] *adj.* 残疾的
27. orthodontic [ˌɔːθəˈdɒntɪk] *adj.* 正畸的；牙齿矫正的
28. interdental cleaning 齿间清洁
29. dental floss 牙线
30. dental tape 洁牙带
31. interdental brushes 牙间隙刷

32. toothpick [ˈtuːθpɪk] *n.* 牙签

33. powered irrigation devices 动力灌洗装置

34. papilla gingiva 牙龈乳头

35. groove [gruːv] *n.* 沟槽

36. gingival margin 龈缘

37. inflammation [ˌɪnfləˈmeɪʃn] *n.* 炎症

38. mouth rinse 漱口水

39. chlorhexidine gluconate 葡萄糖酸氯己定

40. chlorhexidine [klɔːˈheksɪdaɪn] *n.* 氯己定；洗必泰

41. dicationic [dɪˈkeɪʃnɪk] *adj.* 双阳离子的

42. bisbiguanide [bɪsbɪgwˈɑːnɪd] *n.* 双胍类化合物

43. mucositis [ˈmjuːkɒsaɪtɪs] *n.* 黏膜炎

44. epithelial [ˌepɪˈθiːlɪəl] *adj.* 上皮的

45. desquamation [ˌdeskwəˈmeɪʃən] *n.* 脱落；脱屑

46. salivary gland 唾液腺

47. supragingival calculus 龈上结石

48. quaternary ammonium compounds 季铵类化合物

49. cetylpyridinium chloride 西吡氯铵

50. phenolic compounds 酚类化合物

51. zinc citrate 柠檬酸锌

52. polyvinyl methyl ethyl maleic acid 聚乙烯甲基乙基马来酸

53. essential oils 精油

54. mucosa [mjuːˈkəʊsə] *n.* 黏膜

55. stannous fluoride 氟化亚锡

56. oxygenating [ˈɒksɪdʒəneɪtɪŋ] *v.* 给……供氧

57. detergent [dɪˈtɜːdʒənt] *n.* 洗涤剂；去污剂

58. amine alcohols 氨基醇

59. sodium chlorite 次氯酸钠

📝 Notes

❶ The caries process is multifactorial and dynamic and it is possible to arrest or reverse early lesions before cavitation occurs.

龋病是多因素影响的动态过程，在龋洞形成之前有可能阻止或逆转早期病变。

❷ There are two broad approaches to caries control：（1）strengthening or protecting the tooth and （2） behavior modification to reduce the availability of substrate and to promote the regular removal of plaque.

控制龋病有两种主要途径：(1)加强或保护牙齿；(2)行为改变以减少基质的可用性并促进牙菌斑的定期清除。

❸ Regular disturbance of the biofilm by toothbrushing prevents plaque accumulation and is the principal vehicle for introducing fluoride to teeth.

刷牙对生物膜的定期破坏可以防止牙菌斑的积聚，并且是将氟化物作用于牙齿的主要途径。

❹ It has several anticaries properties but the principal action when present in plaque fluid is to promote remineralization over demineralization in the caries process.

氟化物有几种防龋特性，但当存在于牙菌斑液中时，其主要作用是促进龋齿的再矿化而不是脱矿化。

❺ Swallowing and eating toothpaste during dental development can lead to mottling （fluorosis）, which in severe cases can be unaesthetic. Acute overdose can also occur if fluoride ingestion is excessive, leading to systemic toxicity at doses of 1 mg/kg or even death if doses exceed 5 mg/kg.

在牙齿发育期间吞咽和食用牙膏会导致牙齿呈现斑块(氟中毒)，在严重情况下牙齿是不美观的。如果氟摄入过量，也可能发生急性药物过量情况，在剂量为 1 mg/kg时导致全身毒性，如果剂量超过 5 mg/kg 甚至会导致死亡。

❻ Xylitol is an artificial sweetener commonly used as a replacement for sugar. Xylitol is non-acidogenic and has anticaries properties due to antimicrobial actions.

木糖醇是一种人工甜味剂，通常用作糖的替代品。木糖醇不产酸，因其抗菌作用而具有防龋特性。

❼ Clinical guidelines aid treatment planning based on an individual's caries risk assessment. The interval for dental recall should also be linked to a patient's risk status so those at high risk of caries are recalled more frequently for examination and preventive care.

临床指导方针有助于根据个人的龋齿风险评估制定治疗计划。在复诊的间隔时间也应与患者的风险状况相联系，以便让那些龋齿风险较高的人更频繁地被召回进行检查和预防性护理。

❽ Professional actions are also only relevant to those people regularly accessing dental care. For this reason, partnership working and the use of multidisciplinary teams are vital to engaging communities to reduce risk factors for caries.

专业性措施也只与那些定期接受牙科护理的人有关。因此，合作伙伴关系和使用多学科团队对于让社区参与减少龋齿风险因素来说至关重要。

❾ A medium-filament small flat-headed brush is recommended and some authorities recommend changing the toothbrush every 3 months, although there is no evidence that this is critical to plaque removal.

建议使用中等细丝的小平头牙刷，一些权威人士建议每 3 个月更换一次牙刷，尽管没有证据表明这对去除菌斑至关重要。

❿ In clinical studies, toothbrushing alone has been shown to remove between 39% and 50% of plaque and to result in a 35% reduction in gingival bleeding.

临床研究表明，仅刷牙一项就可清除 39%~50% 的菌斑，减少 35% 的牙龈出血。

⓫ Patients with limited manual dexterity, those caring for mentally handicapped patients, or orthodontic patients could consider a powered brush. Powered brushes have also been shown to enhance long-term compliance and so might be suitable for patients who are unable to achieve good plaque control using a manual brush.

手部灵活度有限的患者、照顾智障患者的人或正畸患者可以考虑使用电动牙刷。电动牙刷已被证明可提高长期依从性，因此可能适用于使用手动刷牙无法很好控制牙菌斑的患者。

⓬ Studies have shown that the addition of interdental cleaning reduces bleeding on probing by 67% compared with 35% using toothbrushing alone. Interdental plaque should be removed at 12 to 48-hour intervals so daily interdental cleaning is therefore recommended.

研究表明，与单纯刷牙的 35% 相比，刷牙配合牙间隙清洁可减少 67% 的探诊出血。牙间隙处的菌斑应每隔 12 至 48 小时清除一次，因此建议每天进行牙间隙清洁。

⑬ Chlorhexidine was the earliest and one of the most effective antiplaque agents available. It is a dicationic bisbiguanide available in 0.12% and 0.2% preparations for twice daily use.

氯己定作为一种双胍类药物是最早且最有效的抗菌斑剂之一，有0.12%和0.2%的制剂可供每日两次使用。

⑭ Stannous fluoride has been shown to reduce gingival inflammation and bleeding, although it has less of an effect on plaque levels. It is possible that it exerts its anti-inflammatory effect through modifying the plaque rather than removing it.

氟化亚锡已被证明可以减少牙龈炎症和出血，尽管它对菌斑水平的影响较小。氟化亚锡可能通过修饰菌斑而不是清除菌斑来发挥抗炎作用。

（本单元由杜民权选编）

（文字部分选自 *Dentistry at a Glance*，1st Edition，Part 2，Chapters 22 and 23）

Unit 15 ▶ Prevention of Periodontal Disease

1. General Remarks

The pathogenesis of periodontitis is multifactorial. Theoretically, if we could intervene at any level of the causal pathway, then we could reduce the burden of periodontitis to individuals and society. Despite much investigation, only a few of these risk factors are currently modifiable in order to prevent the occurrence of disease.

2. Microbial Complexes

Bacteria are present on teeth in microcolonies within an amorphous mass of biofilm known as dental plaque. Dental plaque is the main aetiological factor in the development of gingivitis and periodontitis.

2.1 Gingivitis

There is good evidence that chronic gingivitis does not occur in the absence of plaque, and when plaque accumulates, gingivitis almost invariably develops. Removal of plaque has been shown to lead to resolution of experimentally induced gingivitis in all cases. Chronic gingivitis can be prevented by meticulous self-performed plaque removal and chemical plaque control.

本单元正文内容选自 Elizabeth Kay 所著 *Dentistry at a Glance*, John Wiley & Sons, Inc., 2016, Chapter 24, pp.52-53, 选用时已删除所有图片。

2.2   Periodontitis

Periodontitis is a chronic inflammatory disease caused by inflammation of the supporting tissues around the teeth. The infection begins with a microbial shift within the dental plaque from Gram-positive bacteria, which are compatible with periodontal health, to a dysbiotic biofilm characterized predominately by Gram-negative anaerobes and spirochaetes. This pathogenic biofilm induces an inflammatory response that can lead to the formation of periodontal pockets and the destruction of alveolar bone and periodontal ligament.

3.   Primary Prevention

Animal studies have established that clinical attachment loss occurs at sites of plaque accumulation over time, although some animals were resistant to periodontitis despite the presence of plaque. In humans, periodontitis occurs interproximally in areas of plaque accumulation and on teeth where plaque removal is more difficult. In one deprived population without access to dental treatment and who did not practise regular toothbrushing, periodontitis occurred in all of the subjects although there was wide variation in the extent and severity of attachment loss. In patients who have low levels of plaque and gingival inflammation, the development and progression of periodontitis is rare. Periodontitis is a complex multifactorial disease associated with multiple risk factors but dental plaque is necessary, although not on its own sufficient, to cause severe periodontitis. The daily removal and inhibition of the biofilm is key to the primary prevention of periodontitis [1].

4.   Secondary Prevention

Although plaque formation happens relatively quickly after toothbrushing or polishing, the re-infection of periodontal pockets takes longer to occur. Once periodontal health has been established it has been shown that in the absence of optimal oral hygiene measures it can still take months for a periodontopathic biofilm to be re-established on the root surface [2]. It is the prevention of the formation of this mature subgingival plaque that is essential for periodontal health.

Once periodontal treatment is complete, periodontal health can be maintained for many years if patients continue to practice excellent oral hygiene and comply with a supportive periodontal care regime. Recurrence is common among those who do not.

Needs-based professionally performed supportive care and prophylaxis, including monitoring of plaque levels, plaque removal, and targeted oral hygiene advice, has been shown to reduce periodontal bone loss to negligible levels. Three-monthly visits seem to be an optimal time interval for professional care [3].

5. Smoking

Smoking has been shown to be associated with an increased risk of periodontal disease, which increases depending on the frequency and duration of the habit (risk ratio 3.25-7.28) [4]. It is estimated that smoking accounts for 50%-80% of all periodontal diseases. Patients who smoke have also been shown to be more resistant to treatment and are more likely to see recurrence and progression of their periodontal disease after it has been treated. Smoking is also an independent risk factor for tooth loss in patients with treated periodontitis and smoking cessation has been shown to be associated with better periodontal outcomes. 8136A339

Strategies to prevent periodontal disease should include avoiding smoking and providing smoking cessation advice for smokers. Dental professionals should ask all patients about their smoking habits and should advise them of the effects of the periodontium [5]. Patients with periodontitis should either be given a brief intervention from the dentist or referred to the appropriate service.

6. Local Factors

Gingivitis and periodontitis can be caused by subgingival restoration margins and poorly contoured restorations that are plaque retentive. Care and attention in the contouring of interproximal restoration and ensuring an excellent marginal fit of all indirect restoration will minimize their periodontal effects [6]. Partial dentures also contribute to periodontitis and care should be taken in the design of dentures to enable cleaning, minimize gingival coverage, and maximize tooth support to mitigate against this effect.

7. Other Measures

Periodontitis is associated with obesity, diabetes, stress nutritional deficiency, and deprivation, as well as other systemic factors. Taking a holistic approach to general health measures to ensure good systemic health, including a healthy balanced diet, maintaining a healthy weight, maintaining normoglycemia, and measures to address social inequalities, should have an overall effect of reducing periodontal diseases [7].

8. Challenges

One of the challenges in the reduction of plaque is the compliance of patients with suggested oral hygiene regimes. There are patient groups for whom compliance is difficult or impossible, including those with a mental or physical disability. In the general population, oral hygiene is poor and the use of interdental aids, including floss, is low. In the UK, 62% of patients who opted to brush their teeth immediately prior to examination still had visible plaque. Just under a quarter of all teeth in the study had visible plaque.

Public health funding must be in place to ensure training and remuneration of the dental team are adequate and that appropriate educational and motivational strategies are applied at both a population and individual level.

Word List

1. pathogenesis [ˌpæθəˈdʒenɪsɪs] *n.* 发病机理
2. intervene [ˌɪntəˈviːn] *v.* 干预；干涉
3. modifiable [ˈmɒdɪfaɪəbl] *adj.* 可修饰的
4. microcoloniy [maɪkˈrɒkələnɪ] *n.* 微小菌落
5. aetiological [iːtɪəˈlɒdʒɪkəl] *adj.* 病因论的
6. chronic gingivitis 慢性龈炎
7. Gram-positive bacteria 革兰氏阳性菌
8. Gram-negative bacteria 革兰氏阴性菌
9. dysbiotic biofilm 失调的生物膜
10. predominately [prɪˈdɒmɪnətlɪ] *adv.* 占优势地
11. anaerobes [æˈneərəubz] *n.* 厌氧菌
12. spirochaetes [spɪərəˈtʃiːts] *n.* 螺旋体
13. accumulation [əˌkjuːmjəˈleɪʃn] *n.* 堆积；积聚
14. attachment loss 附着丧失

15. oral hygiene measure 口腔卫生措施

16. periodontopathic [ˌperɪədɒntəˈpæθɪk] *adj.* 导致牙周疾病的

17. subgingival plaque 龈下菌斑

18. supportive periodontal care regime 支持性牙周护理方案

19. negligible [ˈneglɪdʒəbl] *adj.* 可忽略不计的

20. periodontium [ˌperiəˈdɒnʃɪəm] *n.* 牙周组织

21. contouring [kənˈtuərɪŋ] *n.* 轮廓线

22. partial dentures 局部义齿

23. obesity [əʊˈbiːsətɪ] *n.* 过度肥胖；肥胖症

24. diabetes [ˌdaɪəˈbiːtiːz] *n.* 糖尿病

25. nutritional deficiency 营养不良

26. deprivation [ˌdeprɪˈveɪʃn] *n.* 匮乏；剥夺

27. holistic [həʊˈlɪstɪk] *adj.* 整体的；全面的

28. normoglycemia [ˌnɔːməʊglaɪˈsiːmɪə] *n.* 血糖正常

29. social inequalities 社会不平等

30. compliance [kəmˈplaɪəns] *n.* 依从性

31. public health funding 公共卫生资金

📝 Notes

❶ Periodontitis is a complex multifactorial disease associated with multiple risk factors but dental plaque is necessary, although not on its own sufficient, to cause severe periodontitis. The daily removal and inhibition of the biofilm is key to the primary prevention of periodontitis.

牙周炎是一种复杂的多因素疾病，与多种危险因素相关，其中牙菌斑是导致重度牙周炎的必要条件。日常清除和抑制生物膜是牙周炎一级预防的关键。

❷ Although plaque formation happens relatively quickly after toothbrushing or polishing, the re-infection of periodontal pockets takes longer to occur. Once periodontal health has been established it has been shown that in the absence of optimal oral hygiene measures it can still take months for a periodontopathic biofilm to be re-established on the root surface.

虽然牙菌斑在刷牙或抛光后的形成相对较快，但牙周袋的再次感染需要更长的时间。有研究表明，一旦建立了牙周健康状态，即使在缺乏最佳口腔卫生措施的情况下，牙周致病性生物膜仍需要数月时间才能在牙根表面重新形成。

❸ Needs-based professionally performed supportive care and prophylaxis, including monitoring of plaque levels, plaque removal, and targeted oral hygiene advice, has been shown to reduce periodontal bone loss to negligible levels. Three-monthly visits seem to be an optimal time interval for professional care.

研究表明，基于专业人员实施的支持性护理和预防措施，包括菌斑水平监测、菌斑清除和针对性的口腔卫生指导，能将牙周骨丧失降低到可忽略不计的水平。每三个月进行一次口腔专业护理似乎是最佳的就诊间隔。

❹ Smoking has been shown to be associated with an increased risk of periodontal disease, which increases depending on the frequency and duration of the habit (risk ratio 3.25-7.28).

吸烟已被证明与牙周病风险增加相关，牙周病风险的增加取决于吸烟的频率和持续时间(风险比 3.25~7.28)。

❺ Strategies to prevent periodontal disease should include avoiding smoking and providing smoking cessation advice for smokers. Dental professionals should ask all patients about their smoking habits and should advise them of the effects of the periodontium.

预防牙周病的策略应包括避免吸烟和向吸烟的人提供戒烟建议。牙科专业人员应询问所有患者的吸烟习惯，并告知他们吸烟对牙周组织的影响。

❻ Gingivitis and periodontitis can be caused by subgingival restoration margins and poorly contoured restorations that are plaque retentive. Care and attention in the contouring of interproximal restoration and ensuring an excellent marginal fit of all indirect restoration will minimize their periodontal effects.

牙龈炎和牙周炎可能是由龈下修复体边缘和轮廓不佳导致菌斑滞留引起的。小心谨慎地制作修复体的邻面轮廓，并确保所有间接修复体的边缘贴合良好，可以最大限度地减少对牙周的影响。

❼ Periodontitis is associated with obesity, diabetes, stress nutritional deficiency, and deprivation, as well as other systemic factors. Taking a holistic approach to general health measures to ensure good systemic health, including a healthy balanced diet, maintaining a healthy weight, maintaining normoglycemia, and measures to address social inequalities, should have an overall effect of reducing periodontal diseases.

牙周炎与肥胖、糖尿病、压力、营养缺乏和匮乏以及其他系统性因素密切相关。采取全面的常规的保健措施确保良好的全身健康，包括健康的均衡饮食、保持健康的体重、维持正常的血糖以及解决社会不平等问题的措施，应能从整体上减少牙周疾病。

（本单元由杜民权选编）

（文字部分选自 *Dentistry at a Glance*, 1st Edition, Part 2, Chapter 24）

Unit 16 ▸ Crowns and Bridges

1. Introduction

Definition: A crown is an extracoronal dental restoration that covers the outer surface of the clinical crown and reproduces the clinical crown of a natural tooth [1].

The crown is cemented onto the prepared clinical crown to aid in its protection, restore its function and dental appearance.

1.1 Types of Crowns

a. **Full crown** : covers all surfaces of the clinical crown of the tooth.

b. **Partial crown** : covers most but not all available surfaces of the clinical crown of the tooth. Typically, most of the buccal surface is left uncovered. Common designs include three-quarter and seven-eighth crowns.

c. **Surveyed crown** : full crown for an abutment tooth for a removable partial denture, which incorporates design features intended to aid in the support and retention for the partial denture [2]. Common incorporates design features of surveyed crowns include undercuts, guide planes and one or more rest seat recesses whilst the definitive crown restoration is being constructed.

d. **Implant-retained crown** : a cement or screw-retained crown fitted over an implant abutment. It derives its support from the implant abutment and underlying implant.

e. **Temporary crown** : preformed or customised crown placed as an interim restoration

本单元正文内容选自 Elizabeth Kay 所著 *Dentistry at a Glance*, John Wiley & Sons, Inc., 2016, Chapters 50 and 53, pp.106-108, pp.112-113, 选用时图表序号有变动。

on prepared teeth. The former is usually made of polycarbonate or aluminium, whereas the latter requires an impression taken prior to tooth preparation. The functions of temporary crowns include: protection of exposed dentine following tooth preparation, maintenance of proximal and occlusal contacts, prevention of overeruption of opposing tooth, and maintenance of function and appearance whilst the definitive crown restoration is being constructed.

1.2 General Indications for Crowns

a. Replacement of a large filling when there is not sufficient tooth tissue remaining for an other intracoronal restoration.

b. Restoration of a fractured or cracked tooth.

c. Protection of a weak tooth from fracturing.

d. In situations of heavy occlusal loading where tooth could potentially fracture.

e. Cover a (usually posterior) tooth that has had root canal treatment and when an onlay is not indicated.

f. Cover a severely discoloured or poorly shaped tooth.

g. Restoration of a single dental implant.

1.3 General Contraindications

a. Evidence of active caries, endodontic or periodontal disease.

b. Aesthetics (metallic crowns).

c. Economic factors.

d. Where patient management requires short visits and simple procedures.

2. Materials for Crown

2.1 Metallic Crown

Cast gold alloy crown is prepared from alloys of various metallic constituents, including but not limited to gold, platinum, palladium, silver, copper and tin (Figure 16.1a).

2.1.1 Advantages

Excellent wear resistance, does not cause wear of opposing teeth, anatomy of tooth can readily be reproduced in the wax prior to casting, can be used in thin section, excellent longevity, and less tooth reduction required than for metal-ceramic and all-ceramic restorations.

2.1.2 Disadvantages

Not aesthetic, cost of alloy.

2.1.3 Preparation Features

a. 1.5 mm occlusal clearance over functional (supporting) cusps and 1 mm clearance of non-functional cusps.

b. Functional cusp bevel.

c. 5°-16° circumferential taper, 0.8-1 mm chamfer margin removing all undercut areas.

d. Should finish supragingivally; this may not always be possible as preparation should extend more gingivally than existing restoration so that the preparation margin finishes on tooth structure.

2.2 Metal-ceramic Crown

Metal-ceramic crown (also known as porcelain-fused-to-metal or bonded crown) combine both the exceptional aesthetic properties of ceramics and the extraordinary mechanical properties of metals. Metal-ceramic crown has a metal subframe to which the porcelain is added in layers. The inner opaque porcelains are added to mask the metal and over this aesthetic porcelains are added to produce the shape and shade of the crown. Metal-ceramic crown may have occlusal ceramic coverage (Figure 16.1b) or occlusal metal coverage (Figure 16.1c). The junction between metal and ceramic should not be in areas of high occlusal stress, as this might result in stress concentration areas with subsequent chipping of the ceramic at the interface.

2.2.1 Advantages

Aesthetics, strength.

2.2.2 Disadvantages

Relatively heavy tooth preparation is required to accommodate the metal and ceramic, potentially resulting in weakening the remaining tooth structure. In addition, ceramic occlusal surfaces may result in wear of opposing tooth surfaces, as ceramic is

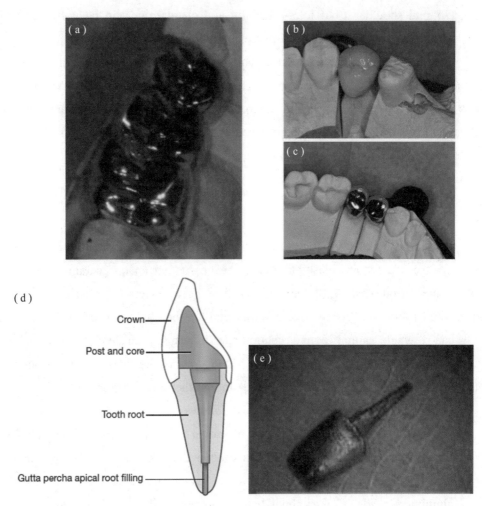

Figure 16.1　（a）Example of full coverage gold alloy crowns on a model；（b）Metal-ceramic crown with ceramic occlusal coverage；（c）Metal-ceramic crowns with metal occlusal coverage；（d）Schematic illustration of a post-retained crown；（e）Cast gold post and core.

（选自 *Dentistry at a Glance*，1st Edition，Part 2，Chapter 50，Figures 50.1-50.5）

more abrasive than enamel. The aesthetics of metal-ceramic crowns may not match those of all-ceramic crowns.

2.2.3　Preparation Features

a. Minimum 1.5 mm reduction for all porcelain fused to metal surfaces of the crown.

b. Functional cusp bevel.

c. 1.5 mm axial reduction.

d. 5°-16° circumferential taper.

e. 1.5 mm shoulder (but joint) labially and chamfer margin palatally/ lingually, which need only be shallow if porcelain coverage is partial.

The preparation is more aggressive than for cast gold crowns, but in general less aggressive than for all-ceramic crowns. A less aggressive preparation for metal-ceramic crowns involves full metal coverage of the occlusal surface of the metal-ceramic crown. In addition, unlike with porcelain occlusal coverage, the metal occlusal surface is not abrasive to the opposing natural dentition.

2.3 All-ceramic Crown

Although the cores used for all-ceramic crowns are not made of metal, they are usually opaque and require masking. Thus, the bright and opaque ceramic coping, like metal copings, need masking by the addition of porcelain layers to produce the shape and shade of the final crown. Because there is no metal to block light transmission, all-ceramic crowns can resemble natural tooth structure better in terms of shade and translucency than any other restorative option. As a result, these crowns are increasingly popular with dentists and patients to provide the most pleasing aesthetic restoration.

All-ceramic materials can be classified as follows:

a. **Conventional ceramics**: This type of crown (e.g. Inceram®, Vita Zahnfabrik, Bad Säckingen, Germany) consists of two distinct layers. The strength of the crown is derived from its inner core, which is made from zirconium and aluminium oxide. Conventional low-fusing porcelains are fired onto the core to create an aesthetically pleasing high-compressive-strength restoration.

b. **Pressed ceramics**: An example of a pressed glass ceramic is IPS Empress (Ivoclar®, Vivadent, Schaan, Liechtenstein). It comprises two layers: an inner core material made of lithium disilicate (the ingot) and an outer layer made from fluouroapatite ceramic. The core is made using the lost wax technique. Wax is invested in a phosphate-bonded investment material and following burn-out, the leucite reinforced glass ceramic is pressed under pressure into the space left by the wax.

c. **CAD/CAM without coping**: This type of crown (e.g., Cerec III system) is manufactured by capturing a digital image of the preparation and opposing dentition, using a intraoral optical scanner to capture a 3D image. The software program of the system allows for the preparation margins to be outlined.

Subsequently, the digital data is transmitted to a computer-controlled milling machine, which mills the final restoration from a monochromatic ceramic block. The ceramic crown is usually milled within 20 minutes. Disadvantages of this system include the relatively high cost of the equipment and that the restoration is limited to one shade only. This can restrict the aesthetic outcome of the all-ceramic crown.

d. **CAD/CAM with coping** : An example of a CAD/CAM system with coping is the Procera® crown (Nobel Biocare, Gothenburg, Sweden). Digital impression data is sent, via email, to a central laboratory, then an alumina coping is produced by the Procera® machine. The coping is then returned to the local technician to complete the crown by veneering it with additional layers of conventional porcelain to create the final restoration.

Luting of all-ceramic crown usually consists of bonding the ceramic restoration to the prepared tooth using the acid etch technique and the use of a resin luting cement. Bonding to ceramic is achieved by etching the fit surface with hydrofluoric acid and the use of a silane coupling agent.

2.3.1 Advantages

Superior aesthetics, excellent translucency, high compressive strength, good soft tissue response, i.e. high biocompatibility.

2.3.2 Disadvantages

Brittle, low-tensile strength, shoulder-type margin preparation circumferentially results in significantly more tooth preparation on the palatal/lingual and proximal surfaces than for metal-ceramic crowns.

2.3.3 Indications

Areas with high aesthetic requirement where a more conservative restoration would be inadequate.

2.3.4 Contraindications

When more conservative restorations can be used. All-ceramic crowns are rarely indicated for molars because of the increased occlusal load and reduced aesthetic demand.

3. Post-retained Crown

Posts are used to retain restorations or cores for extracoronal restorations in endodontically treated teeth when there is insufficient tooth tissue to provide retention and support for a restoration [3]. It is important to note that posts do not reinforce roots of weakened, endodontically treated teeth. On the contrary, preparation for a post results in further weakening of the root, potentially predisposing it to root fracture.

3.1   Components

3.1.1   Post

The component that extends into the root canal. Its length should be at least equal to the height of the clinical crown. At least 5 mm of gutta percha must remain apical to the post in order to maintain an adequate apical seal (Figure 16.1d).

3.1.2   Core

The structure connected to the post that supports and retains the crown.

3.1.3   Crown

The component that fits over the core to restore the function and appearance of the tooth.

3.2   Indications

3.2.1   Endodontic Factors

a. Good-quality, symptom-free root filling.

b. Evidence or prospect of periapical healing.

3.2.2   Periodontal Factors

a. Absence of progressive periodontal disease.

b. Alveolar bone sufficient to support the restored tooth in clinical service.

3.2.3   Restorative and Occlusal Factors

a. Sufficient (radicular) tooth tissue remaining to support and retain a post crown.

b. Favourable location and angulation of endodontically treated root relative to the adjacent and opposing teeth.

c. Favourable occlusal relationship to limit loading of the post crown in function.

The success of a post-retained restoration is greatly increased if sufficient coronal tooth tissue remains supragingivally for the availability of a ferrule. The ferrule effect has been described as an encircling band of the cast restoration around the coronal surface of the tooth, which provides bracing and retention.

The presence of a ferrule reduces the stresses at the end of the post, thus reducing the risk of root fracture. The additional support and retention gained by a ferrule reduces the risk of de-bonding of the restoration. Whilst at least 1 mm in height improves fracture resistance, at least 2 mm is considered optimal. The thickness of the axial walls must be at least 1 mm to contribute to the ferrule.

Careful assessment of the endodontically treated tooth is made for the following:

a. Good apical seal.

b. No sensitivity to pressure.

c. No exudates.

d. No fistula.

e. No apical sensitivity.

f. No active inflammation.

Note that an inadequately root filled tooth should be retreated prior to the placement of a new post core.

3.3　Contraindications

a. Carious root surface.

b. Evidence of apical periodontitis.

c. Active periodontal disease.

d. Inadequate alveolar bone support.

e. Root perforations, cracks and fractures.

f. Deep subgingival margins—consider crown lengthening or extrusion.

g. Crown length will exceed remaining root length.

h. Failed endodontic treatment.

i. Insufficient space for final restoration.

3.4　Types of Posts

3.4.1　Active and Passive Posts

Active posts are usually prefabricated and threaded in design, and can either be self-threading or pretapped. When placing a self-threading post, the thread of the post cuts the counter thread into the walls of the dentine. The use of active, threaded posts, is associated with increased stresses and root fracture; particularly with a tapered design resulting in an additional 'wedging' effect into the post space [4]. Pretapped post systems use a pretapping device to cut the counter thread into the dentine walls prior to post cementation.

Whilst active posts are more retentive than passive posts of similar dimensions, the latter are often preferred, as less strain is introduced into the root, thus reducing the risk of root fracture. Passive posts can either be custom-made (i.e., cast post and core) or prefabricated. Their surface is usually either smooth or serrated, and their shape can be either tapered or parallel. In general, parallel-sided, serrated posts are the most retentive types of passive posts.

3.4.2   Metallic and Non-metal Posts:

Custom-made cast posts and cores (indirect, laboratory made) are most commonly made from precious metal alloys (Figure 16.1e), whilst prefabricated metallic posts are commonly made from stainless steel, titanium alloy, nickel-chrome or other non-precious metal alloys. An advantage of metallic posts is their strength and radiopacity (Table 16.1). A potential disadvantage of using non-precious metal alloy posts is their tendency to undergo corrosion.

The more recent, non-metallic posts are made out of either carbon, silica or quartz fibres embedded longitudinally in an epoxy resin, or zirconia. These are more radiolucent than the metal alternatives and rely on resin based luting cements.

Table 16.1   Comparison of Metallic and Non-metallic Posts

Metallic posts		Non-metallic posts	
Advantages	Disadvantages	Advantages	Disadvantages
Radiopaque	Increased risk of vertical root fracture (due to direct transmission of occlusal forces to root dentine)	Microscopic flexure (modulus of elasticity is similar to dentine)	Radiolucent
Good strength	Corrosion (only non-precious alloys)	Aesthetics (posts are translucent, white or tooth-coloured)	If resin luting cement failure occurs then it is usually partial and does not result in complete debonding (decementation) of the post; thus allowing ingress of saliva and bacteria into radicular dentine (where partial debonding has occurred) resulting in extensive decay and catastrophic failure of the remaining tooth.

(选自 *Dentistry at a Glance*, 1st Edition, Part 2, Chapter 50, Table 50.1)

4.   Introduction

Definition: A bridge is a dental prosthesis used to replace a missing tooth or teeth. It typically cannot be removed by the patient [5].

The components of a bridge include:

a. Retainer: part of bridge that is fitted to the abutment tooth.

b. Pontic: artificial tooth that replaces the missing natural tooth or teeth.

c. Connector: the element of the bridge that joins the pontic to the retainer; the connector may be rigid or movable.

Further relevant terms include:

a. Unit: a term used to indicate the number of pontics and retainers associated with the bridge; for example, a three-unit bridge = two retainers + one pontic.

b. Pier abutment: a non-terminal abutment tooth incorporated in bridge and is commonly the weak link in the bridge design, particularly with long bridges. Bridges can be broadly classified as follows: conventional, resin-bonded (=resin retained or adhesive), hybrid.

5. Conventional Bridges

5.1　Fixed-fixed Design

A retainer is at both ends of the edentulous span; pontic(s) lie between retainers; rigid connector joins pontic to retainers; three or more units (Figure 16.2).

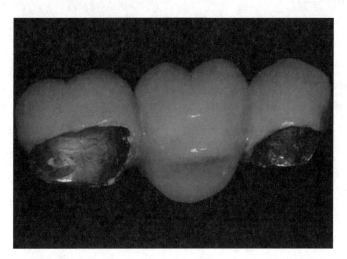

Figure 16.2　Example of a conventional fixed-fixed three-unit bridge replacing UL2
(选自 *Dentistry at a Glance*, 1st Edition, Part 2, Chapter 53, Figure 53.1)

5.1.1　Advantages:

a. Robust design for maximum strength and retention.

b. Splinting of abutment teeth may be advantageous in a patient with stable periodontal disease.

c. Laboratory construction is relatively uncomplicated.

5.1.2 Disadvantages:

a. Extensive tooth preparation of abutment teeth is required.

b. Paralleling the preparations can be difficult if they are widely separated.

c. May experience cementation difficulties as the bridge must be inserted in one piece.

d. Design is not suitable for abutment teeth that are markedly tilted.

5.2 Fixed-movable Design

Utilises a custom-made or proprietary precision attachment to allow a degree of movement between two component parts of the bridge. Typically, on its mesial aspect the pontic is connected, via a movable connector, to the distal end of the mesial retainer. On its distal aspect the pontic is usually connected rigidly to the distal retainer; thereby allowing limited predominantly vertical movement between the pontic and the retainer to which it is linked via the movable connector.

5.2.1 Advantages:

a. Can be used when abutment teeth are divergent.

b. Allows a limited degree of tooth movement.

c. Allows cementation of the bridge in two stages.

5.2.2 Disadvantages:

a. Length of the span is limited to one or two pontics, especially if teeth have some mobility.

b. Laboratory construction is complicated and costly due to incorporation of intracoronal movable component.

c. Difficult to construct a temporary bridge.

5.3 Cantilever Design

The pontic is connected to the retainer(s) at one end only.

5.3.1 Advantages:

a. Preparation of only one abutment tooth is required.

b. Involves one retainer only.

c. No need for paralleling of multiple abutments.

d. Laboratory construction is relatively uncomplicated.

5.3.2   Disadvantages:

a. Leverage forces on the abutment tooth.

b. Torquing forces must not act on the pontic.

6. Resin-bonded Bridges

A fixed prosthesis that is adhesively bonded to one or more unprepared (or minimally prepared) natural teeth and which replaces one or more missing teeth. Resin-bonded bridges are useful for tooth replacement anteriorly (Figure 16.3) and posteriorly (Figure 16.4).

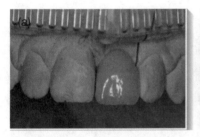 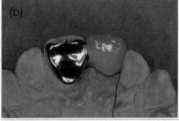 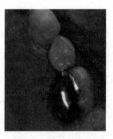

Figure 16.3   (Left) Example of an anterior cantilever resin-retained bridge: (a) frontal view and (b) palatal view.

Figure 16.4   (Right) Example of a posterior cantilever resin-retained bridge.

(选自 *Dentistry at a Glance*, 1st Edition, Part 2, Chapter 53, Figures 53.2 and 53.3)

6.1   Advantages

a. Fixed prosthesis.

b. Conservative of tooth structure.

c. Suitable for use in adolescent patients.

d. Usually does not require local a naesthesia.

e. Limited clinical time required to complete.

f. Relatively inexpensive.

g. Potentially reversible.

h. Good longevity (>80% survival over 10 years).

i. Possible diagnostic precursor to conventional bridgework.

6.2　Disadvantages

a. Sometimes 'greying' shine through appearance of abutment tooth/teeth may be seen from frontal view. However, this can be usually overcome by the use of an opaque luting cement.
b. Risk of debonding (but recementation is usually possible).
c. Longevity is less than for conventional bridgework.
d. Risk of caries is greater in the case of partial debond in the fixed-fixed design (note: a cantilever design overcomes this problem and is the preferred option, whenever possible).

6.3　Indications

a. Ideally, single-tooth replacement using cantilever design (note: fixed-fixed resin-bonded bridges with several pontics have been shown to have a significantly increased debond rate).
b. Sound or minimally restored abutment teeth with sufficient, good-quality enamel for bonding.
c. Intermediate prostheses in young patients during growth phase and prior to implant placement.

6.4　Contraindications

a. Heavily restored abutment teeth.
b. Teeth with short clinical crowns.
c. Abutment teeth damaged by wear.
d. Presence of unstable periodontal disease.
e. Occlusal parafunction.
f. Difficulty in achieving a dry operating field for cementation.
g. Very translucent incisal edges (anterior teeth) because of likelihood of metal shine through appearance. However, this can be counteracted by the application of composite resin restorative materials.

Note: when designing posterior resin-bonded bridges it is essential to wrap the metal wing retainer at least half-way onto the occlusal surface of the abutment tooth for the bridge to adequately withstand shear forces.

7. Hybrid Bridges

Hybrid bridges consist of a combination of a conventional retainer and an adhesive retainer on the terminal abutment teeth [6]. It is advisable to incorporate a movable joint into the design to allow for differential movement between the component of the bridge attached via the conventional retainer on one side and the component attached via the adhesive metal wing retainer on the other side (Figure 16.5a-d). Cementation of the bridge involves the use of conventional cement for the conventional retainer and an adhesive resin-based cement for the adhesive retainer.

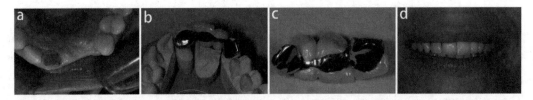

Figure 16.5　(a) UL1 and UL2 missing. Note: UR1 has been previously prepared for a PFM retainer and UL3 is sound. (b) Hybrid bridge with conventional retainer UR1 and adhesive retainer wing on UL3. (c) Movable joint connector between UR1 conventional retainer and UL1 pontic. (d) Hybrid bridge *in situ*.

（选自 *Dentistry at a Glance*, 1st Edition, Part 2, Chapter 53, Figure 53.4）

7.1　Advantages

a. Fixed prosthesis.
b. Preserves tooth tissue by using an adhesive wing retainer for one of the abutments.

7.2　Disadvantages

a. Failure rate is higher than conventional bridgework.
b. Risk of caries is greater in the case of partial debond.

8. Pontic Design for Bridges

Bridge pontic designs include:
a. Ridge lap pontic.
b. Modifed ridge lap pontic.

c. Ovate pontics.

d. Bullet-nose pontic.

e. Sanitary pontic.

The ridge lap pontic closely adapts to, and covers a relatively wide area of, the underlying alveolar ridge. This extensive coverage makes it difficult to clean under the pontic and often leads to inflammation of the area in contact with the pontic. Hence, this type of pontic is unfavourable and should be avoided.

The modified ridge lap pontic is designed to further reduce tissue contact with the underlying ridge. Tissue contact is limited to the labial/buccal surface of the ridge crest, resulting in less tissue irritation than ridge lap pontics. A modified ridge lap pontic allows good cleaning with maximum aesthetics by overlying part of the ridge to mimic emergence of the pontic from the gingival tissues in a similar way to the natural tooth [7].

Ovate pontics may be used in cases where the residual ridge has a localised defect or has incompletely healed. They can also be used in broad and fat ridges. The design of the pontic is such that its cervical end extends into the defect of the edentulous alveolar ridge. The ovate pontic provides an aesthetically pleasing appearance, as it appears to emerge from the ridge like a natural tooth.

Sanitary and bullet-nose pontics are preferred posteriorly where aesthetics is of less concern. This pontic has no tissue contact with the underlying alveolar ridge, which facilitates cleaning under the pontic.

📋 Word List

1. restoration [ˌrestəˈreɪʃn] *n.* 修复体
2. full crown 全冠
3. partial crown 部分冠
4. surveyed crown 观测线冠
5. implant-retained crown 种植牙冠
6. temporary crown 暂时冠
7. definitive crown 最终冠
8. extracoronal [ˌekstrəˈkɒrəʊnəl] *adj.* 冠外的
9. intracoronal [ˌɪntrəˈkɒrəʊnəl] *adj.* 冠内的
10. tooth preparation 牙体预备
11. occlusal loading 咬合负荷
12. metallic crown 金属冠

13. cast [kɑːst] *v.* 铸造

14. metal-ceramic crown 金属烤瓷冠

15. all-ceramic crown 全瓷冠

16. CAD/CAM 计算机辅助设计/计算机辅助制造

17. intraoral optical scanner 口内光学扫描仪

18. digital impression 数字化印模

19. coping [ˈkəʊpɪŋ] *n.* 内冠

20. porcelain [ˈpɔːsəlɪn] *n.* 瓷 *adj.* 瓷制的

21. pressed ceramic 铸瓷

22. mill [mɪl] *v.* 切削；研磨

23. post-retained crown 桩冠

24. core [kɔː(r)] *n.* 核

25. prefabricated [priːˈfæbrɪkeɪtɪd] *adj.* 预制的

26. self-threading [selfˈθredɪŋ] *adj.* 自攻螺纹的

27. cement [sɪˈment] *n.* 水门汀

28. leucite [ˈluːsaɪt] *n.* 白榴石

29. zirconia [zəˈkəʊnɪə] *n.* 氧化锆

30. custom-made cast post 个性化铸造桩

31. pontic [ˈpɒntɪk] *n.* 桥体

32. retainer [rɪˈteɪnə(r)] *n.* 固位体

33. connector [kəˈnektə(r)] *n.* 连接体

34. pier abutment 中间基牙

35. fixed-fixed bridge 双端固定桥

36. fixed-movable bridge 固定-活动桥

37. divergent [daɪˈvɜːdʒənt] *adj.* 分散的

38. cantilever bridge 单端固定桥；悬臂固定桥

39. leverage force 杠杆力

40. torquing force 扭力

41. resin-bonded bridge 树脂粘接桥

42. hybrid bridge 复合固定桥

43. ridge lap pontic 盖嵴式桥体

44. modified ridge lap pontic 改良盖嵴式桥体

45. ovate pontic 卵圆形桥体

46. sanitary pontic 卫生桥体；悬空式桥体

47. alveolar ridge 牙槽嵴

📝 Notes

❶ A crown is an extracoronal dental restoration that covers the outer surface of the clinical crown and reproduces the clinical crown of a natural tooth.
冠是一种覆盖基牙临床牙冠外表面、用来恢复天然牙齿形态和功能的冠外修复体。

❷ Surveyed crown：full crown for an abutment tooth for a removable partial denture, which incorporates design features intended to aid in the support and retention for the partial denture.
观测线冠:为了帮助可摘局部义齿稳定和固位, 在基牙上按照观测线制作的全冠。

❸ Posts are used to retain restorations or cores for extracoronal restorations in endodontically treated teeth when there is insufficient tooth tissue to provide retention and support for a restoration.
对于根管治疗后的牙齿, 仅靠牙体组织不足以为修复体提供足够的固位和支撑时, 就要使用桩来固定修复体或冠外修复体的核。

❹ The use of active, threaded posts, is associated with increased stresses and root fracture; particularly with a tapered design resulting in an additional 'wedging' effect into the post space.
主动螺纹桩的使用与应力增加及根折风险上升紧密相关, 尤其锥形设计的螺纹桩会在桩道中产生额外的"楔入"效应。

❺ A bridge is a dental prosthesis used to replace a missing tooth or teeth. It typically cannot be removed by the patient.
固定桥是一种用来替代单颗或多颗缺失牙的修复体, 患者通常不能自行摘戴。

❻ Hybrid bridges consist of a combination of a conventional retainer and an adhesive retainer on the terminal abutment teeth.
复合固定桥由传统固位体和位于末端基牙上的粘接固位体组合而成。

❼ A modified ridge lap pontic allows good cleaning with maximum aesthetics by overlying part of the ridge to mimic emergence of the pontic from the gingival tissues in a similar way to the natural tooth.

改良盖嵴式桥体通常覆盖部分牙槽嵴(与唇颊侧牙槽嵴顶轻微接触),使得桥体从牙龈组织中以类似天然牙的方式萌出,从而实现了最佳的美学效果和良好的清洁便利性。

(本单元由杨宏业选编)

(文字部分选自 *Dentistry at a Glance*, 1st Edition, Part 2, Chapters 50 and 53)

Unit 17 ▶ Partial Dentures and Complete Dentures

---

1. Partial Dentures

1.1 Introduction

When teeth are lost, there are a variety of options available to the clinician (Figure 17.1a); some of these depend on the patient's oral status, some on her/his motivation and the others depend on ability to meet the potential cost. These options are:

a. Do nothing; leave the space or spaces unrestored.

b. Provide a fixed prosthesis.

c. Provide an implant-supported fixed prosthesis.

d. Provide an implant-supported plus removable partial denture (RPD).

e. Provide a (conventional) RPD.

f. Provide complete denture.

This section will deal with RPDs. There are several types of RPD that may be prescribed and these are listed in Table 17.1, along with some indications for their use. Always remember, however, that RPDs will inevitably serve as plaque-retaining agents and sound advice should be given to the patient on oral hygiene and aftercare.

本单元正文内容选自 Elizabeth Kay 所著 *Dentistry at a Glance*, John Wiley & Sons, Inc., 2016, Chapters 55 and 59, pp.116-117, pp.124-125. 选用时图表序号有改动。

Table 17.1　Types of RPD

Option	Clinical indications
Immediate RPD	To preserve interdental(and interarch space following loss of a tooth or teeth To preserve appearance and phonetics for social reasons
Transitional RPD	May be used in an attempt to raise overdenture or to improve interarch relationships or postinsertion of an implant and prior to integration
Occlusal splint	As used to treat a temporomandibular problem
Definitive RPD	As a planned option to replace missing teeth

(选自 *Dentistry at a Glance*, 1st Edition, Part 2, Chapter 55, Table 55.1)

1.2　Planning Partial Dentures

The stages involved in planning and designing RPDs are listed in Table 17. 2. Following a thorough clinical examination, and after due consultation with the patient, primary impressions should be taken. Depending on the reproducibility and positivity of the retruded contact position (RCP), a primary occlusal registration may also be required. An adequate cast analysis (Figure 17.1b) should be undertaken so that space between the arches for the RPD can be assessed for undercuts and possible guide planes [1].

Table 17.2　Stages in the Design of a RPD

1	Identify and analyse saddles
2	Determine which ones to restore
3	Determine support
4	Join up saddles (major connector)
5	Join supporting elements/retaining elements to major connector
6	Consider indirect retention (Kennedy I, II or IV cases)
7	Reconsider with prevention/maintenance in mind

(选自 *Dentistry at a Glance*, 1st Edition, Part 2, Chapter 55, Box 55.1)

1.3 Sources of Support

Sources of support are listed in Table 17.3. Where only a few teeth remain, mucosal support may well be the only option available. Clinicians should appreciate that, ultimately, such a denture, under occlusal forces, will cause more resorption of the underlying bone and therefore long-term viability and maintenance must be considered [2]. Tooth support is theoretically the optimal option as occlusal forces are directed down the long axes of the teeth, thereby stimulating the periodontal membranes optimally. However, some tooth preparation is likely, for occlusal rests or retaining elements, for example addition of (composite resin) undercuts to retain the denture or to shape guiding surfaces.

Table 17.3　Possible Sources of Support

Source	Descriptor
Mucosa	Least desired as this will tend to accelerate bone loss
Tooth and mucosa	Better than above, but may necessitate planning for antirotational component: the mucosal supporting portion will still promote bone loss, however
Tooth	Best of the 3 conventional options owing to forces being transferred (ideally) down long axis of the teeth may involve tooth via crown or via a root (overdenture)
Implant	Unlikely to have RPD option, but this is possible
Implant and tooth	Popular and better than any option involving mucosal support
Implant and mucosa	Currently popular but rotational movements still possible and therefore a minimum of 3 well-spaced implants will be required

（选自 *Dentistry at a Glance*, 1st Edition, Part 2, Chapter 55, Table 55.2）

1.4 Retention of Dentures

It is incumbent on the clinician to ensure that the denture provided has a retaining element to prevent easy dislodgement from the mouth. There are several ways that this may be provided and these are listed in Table 17.4.

The most common means of retention of a RPD is via a metallic component called a clasp. Basically, this component should engage an undercut and have rigidity to resist distortion yet be sufficient flexibility to slide over the undercut during removal and insertion. A knowledge of the properties of dental alloys is therefore required. Guide planes are surfaces adjacent to saddles, which may be used (and created by selective grinding if required) to resist vertical removal from the mouth. Precision attachments are becoming very popular with implant-supported cases but an awareness of space requirements and aftercare is essential. Indirect retainers are supporting elements that act on the opposite end of the axis of rotation of the denture from the saddle to oppose and hinder rotation [3]. More-flexible materials may be applied to the (freshly cured) denture to engage undercuts between the few remaining teeth and the denture when conventional means of retention is not feasible (Figure 17.1c).

Table 17.4 Possible Sources of Retention of RPDs

Means of retention	Comments
Clasps	Gingivally approaching Occlusally approaching Note, in order to find undercuts into which to direct the clasp tips, surveying is necessary as is a knowledge of the properties of the material chosen
Guide planes	May be used in Kennedy I , II or IV denture designs
Precision attachmenls	Intracoronal Extracoronal Studs Bars Ancillary
Inddirect retainers	For use in tooth and mucosal or implant and mucosal supported RPDs
Other	Silicone rubber to engage undercuts interdentally Denture achesives

（选自 *Dentistry at a Glance*, 1st Edition, Part 2, Chapter 55, Table 55.3）

1.5   Joining the Saddles

This is achieved via major connectors. What we term 'pontics' in fixed bridgework, we term 'major connectors' in RPDs. As can be seen in Table 17.5, there are six types of maxillary major connector and five mandibular types. The type of major connector selected will depend on clinical factors (e. g., status and number of the remaining teeth), anatomical factors (e.g., at least 7.5 mm space is required between the floor of the mouth and the lingual gingival margins of mandibular incisors for a lingual bar and 10.5 mm for a sublingual bar), aesthetic factors (e.g., labial bar may be perceived as unsightly and incisal spacing may preclude metallic anterior bars) and social factors (e.g., anterior bars may affect speech).

Table 17.5   Types of Major Connector

Maxillary	Mandibular
Full palatal coverage	Lingual plate
Palatal plate	Lingual bar
Palatal bar	Sublingual bar
Skeletal design (anterior and posterior palatal bars)	Kennedy bar
Labial bar	Labial bar
Horseshoe	

（选自 *Dentistry at a Glance*, 1st Edition, Part 2, Chapter 55, Table 55.4）

1.6   Completing the Design

Consideration should then be given as to how the supporting and retaining elements are added to the major connector (these are called minor connectors). In simple RPDs they will be incorporated in the acrylic resin denture base. In cobalt chromium dentures, the minor connections will be part of the casting. Thereafter, the denture should be reconsidered along with oral hygiene and patient-related factors, such as the patient's manual dexterity to remove and insert the denture [4]. Always give the patient a leaflet to explain denture care and maintenance.

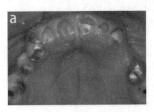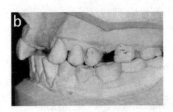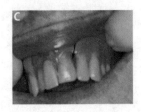

Figure 17.1　(a) Spaces (actual and that caused by decoronation) require consideration for restoration; (b) Articulated casts help visualize spaces available and permit surveying; (c) The retention here is provided by silicone rubber added to the poly (methyl) methacrylate denture base postcuring (arrowed).

(选自 *Dentistry at a Glance*, 1st Edition, Part 2, Chapter 55, Figures 55.1, 55.2 and 55.3)

2. Complete Dentures

2.1　Edentulousness

This clinical condition may arise from neglect, accident or may be hereditary, resulting in anodontia. According to the World Health Organisation, edentulous patients are classified as handicapped and therefore the provision of complete dentures requires an understanding of the underlying science, an appreciation of patient factors and a sound understanding of basic prosthodontic principles.

Table 17.6 lists some of the common features and changes associated with (complete) tooth loss. Resorption affects the residual ridges and this in turn affects extraoral and facial appearance.

Table 17.6　Principal Effects of (Complete) Tooth Loss

Facial changes	Alteration to vertical nasiolabial angle also affects vermillion border Alteration to lip support affects philtrum May, in time, induce a pseudoprognathic appearance
Intraoral changes	Maxilla resorbs inwards, therefore arch becomes more narrow Incisive papilla appears to move anteriorly Mandible appears to widen Residual ridge resorption—this is irrevocable

Continued

Physiological changes	Loss of proprioception from periodonta membrane Reduction of masticatory efficiency Decreased ability to adapt to the edentulous state in older patients, including phonetic problems Need to select appropriate freeway space
Psychological changes	Varies with person to person—may be severe antagonism to loss of teeth May affect confidence
Social changes	Current change in social (non)acceptance of edentulousness Greater emphasis on facial aesthetics

(选自 *Dentistry at a Glance*, 1st Edition, Part 2, Chapter 59, Table 59.1)

Clinicians ought to utilise their knowledge of facial types when prescribing replacement dentures and, further, be aware of the fact that some types; for example Angle's Class 2 div. ii types will tend to lose more bone postextraction, (especially in the mandible) than other types owing to their 90° mandibular angles and a tendency for more prominent masseter muscles.

2.2   Assessing the Patient

When contemplating prescribing replacement dentures, the clinician should be aware of the basic prosthodontic parameters involved, in addition to assessing the patient's wishes and perceptions [5]; if such expectations are unrealistic or beyond your (current) clinical expertise, then common sense should prevail and the patient should be referred to a more senior and experienced colleague. These factors are listed in Table 17.7.

Table 17.7   Basic Aspects to Consider in Planning Complete Dentures (C/Cs)

Factor to consider	Definition	What to watch out for
Support	A feature of the denture-bearing tissues (DBTs) resisting movement of the denture towards these tissues	Assess ability of DBTs to withstand digital pressure Assess nature of DBA (i.e., bony, fibrous) Is DBA inflamed or is there any mucosal pathology present?

Continued

Factor to consider	Definition	What to watch out for
Retention	A feature of the denture periphery resisting movement away from the denture-bearing tissues	Need to provide a peripheral seal Need to determine form and displacability of post dam tissues/ presence of a palatal fissure Assess quality and quantity of saliva
Stability	A feature of the denture resisting anterior-posterior and lateral movements of the denture	All C/Cs require occlusal balance in RCP Check if your patient should have balanced articulation Always ensure that the C/Cs are in harmony with the peridenture musculature(muscle balance) Patient's ability to control denture(s)
Other patient-related factors	Appearance form denture-wearing experience	Establish what the patient wants and (also if this is appropriate!) Inform the patient of the design of the denture—if you plan to leave off some teeth (e.g. 7s), tell the patient why Good denture-wearing history might indicate that replica dentures should be prescribed where indicated and where practicable
Dentist-related factors	Experience laboratory quality Staff experience	Know your limitations! Ensure you have and maintain good communication with your technician Good teamwork is essential for a successful outcome

(选自 *Dentistry at a Glance*, 1st Edition, Part 2, Chapter 59, Table 59.2)

2.3　Prosthodontic Factors

Support: It is essential that the clinician assesses, thoroughly, the denture bearing tissues (DBTs) to determine areas that are unlikely to withstand occlusal loading (e.g. flabby ridges) and which are vulnerable to pressure (e.g. atrophic mucosa, spikey ridges or retained roots; Figure 17.2) [6]. This will also include prescribing an appropriate freeway space (FWS) in older patients with atrophic mandibular ridges—here clinical wisdom would suggest providing a larger FWS to avoid discomfort in mastication. This is the one factor that the clinician should be able to assess accurately and diminish the potential for failure, as retention and stability problems cannot always be overcome.

Retention: Retention requirements mean that the denture need to create a peripheral seal-essentially a triangle incorporating the post dam as the base and the right and left flanges of the upper denture [7]. The presence of a clef palate or a palatal clef (Figure 17.3) can jeopardise a peripheral seal, as can muscle attachments that obliterate the sulcus. Also, absence of saliva will mean that the small but beneficial role of surface tension in the retention of a denture will be impaired.

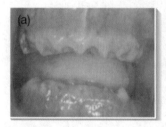 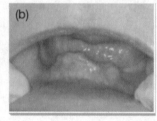 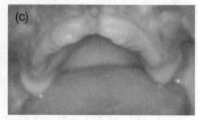

Figure 17.2 Examples of support problems: (a, b) these ealing sockets will present support problems; (c) neither the image nor a study cast will reflect that the anterior ridge is flabby.

(选自 *Dentistry at a Glance*, 1st Edition, Part 2, Chapter 59, Figure 59.1)

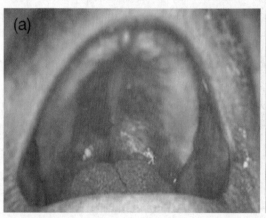 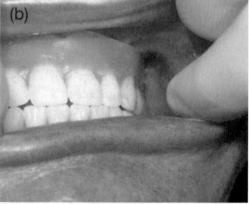

Figure 17.3 Examples of retention problems: (a) a palatal fissure in the post dam area (arrowed); (b) denture flange on the patient's left which, although impinging slightly on the muscle attachment, does not fill the peripheral roll

(选自 *Dentistry at a Glance*, 1st Edition, Part 2, Chapter 59, Figure 59.2)

Stability: This is the most complex and uncertain aspect of complete denture prescription. It is dependent on a combination of occlusal balance (OB), muscle balance (MB) and patient skills; the latter are, in the main, beyond the clinician's ability to control and many dentures have been prescribed which satisfy prosthodontic norms yet fail to gain patient acceptance. The converse is also true. Muscle balance requires care in recording the definitive impressions, while occlusal balance needs assessment at the initial consultation. Clinicians ought to prescribe OB in retruded contact positions (RCPs) for all dentures by ensuring that the registration stage is recorded properly, using specialized techniques if necessary. However, it will not be possible to ensure that balanced articulation can be prescribed. As this is required for stability in for ruminatory movements in eating, and stability problems must be anticipated in most patients.

2.3.1   Other Patient-related Factors

These will include perceptions of how the dentures should look, the number and form of teeth on the denture and denture-wearing experience. A balance must be struck between what is desired and what is feasible. For example, patient preferences for tooth selection may very well have to hold sway against that of the clinician, but in cases where stability indicates that second molars should be left of the denture, then the patient should be made aware of the fact that stability matters have to take precedence. Contentment with a particular form of the denture periphery may well mean that the clinician should opt to prescribe a replica or template denture. In this case the clinician must ensure that the peripheral form is faithfully reproduced and that the occlusal form of the replacement denture does not induce instability as, in most cases, a worn-down occlusal surface will be being replaced by teeth with cusps.

2.3.2   Dentist-related Factors

The art of complete denture prosthodontics is a problem area to younger graduates, who now treat fewer completed denture patients than undergraduates of 20 years ago. As the number of adults who are edentulous falls, undergraduates who are edentulous will become more problematic to treat-yet their expectations of success may very well be raised by virtue of the power of advertising in the media. One consequence of this is that a combination of lack of training allied to fear of failure may mean that many clinicians may fail to inspire patient confidence. In a clinician who is treating a complete denture patient with any lack of this quality, the chances of realistic success are much diminished.

Finally, the provision of complete dentures does require the harmonious integration of the dental team including the clinician, the dental technician/clinical dental technician, the dental surgery assistance and the receptionist [8]. The incorporation of available leaflets with the practice booklet will, in addition, keep the patient informed of what is required, for after care and maintenance.

📝 Word List

1. removable partial denture (RPD) 可摘局部义齿
2. primary impression 初印模
3. retruded contact position (RCP) 后退接触位
4. saddle ['sædl] *n.* 鞍基
5. major connector 大连接体
6. minor connector 小连接体
7. mucosal support 黏膜支持
8. tooth support 牙支持
9. rest [rest] *n.* 支托
10. dislodgement [dɪs'lɒdʒmənt] *n.* 脱位
11. clasp [klɑːsp] *n.* 卡环
12. guide plane 导平面
13. selective grinding 选磨
14. precision attachment 精密附着体
15. denture base 基托
16. acrylic resin 丙烯树脂
17. cobalt chromium 钴铬合金
18. lingual bar 舌杆
19. lingual plate 舌板
20. occlusal registration 咬合记录
21. retention [rɪ'tenʃn] *n.* 固位
22. indirect retainer 间接固位体
23. direct retainer 直接固位体
24. axis of rotation 转动轴；支点线
25. surveying line 观测线
26. occlusal splint 咬合夹板
27. complete denture 全口义齿
28. edentulousness [iː'dentʃələsnɪs] *n.* 无牙颌
29. anodontia [ˌænə'dɒnʃɪə] *n.* 无牙；牙缺失
30. support [sə'pɔːt] *n.* 支持
31. stability [stə'bɪlətɪ] *n.* 稳.定

32. nasolabial angle 鼻唇角
33. arch [ɑːtʃ] *n.* 牙弓
34. proprioception [ˌprəʊprɪəˈsepʃən] *n.* 本体感受
35. denture-bearing tissues (DBTs) 义齿承托组织
36. peripheral seal 边缘封闭
37. occlusal balance (OB) 咬合平衡
38. muscle balance (MB) 肌肉平衡

✍ Notes

❶ An adequate cast analysis should be undertaken so that space between the arches for the RPD can be assessed for undercuts and possible guide planes.
为了准确评估可摘局部义齿的咬合空间是否存在倒凹和潜在的导平面，医生应当进行充分的模型分析。

❷ Clinicians should appreciate that, ultimately, such a denture, under occlusal forces, will cause more resorption of the underlying bone and therefore long-term viability and maintenance must be considered.
医生应当认识到，在咬合力的长期作用下，可摘局部义齿将加剧牙槽骨的吸收，因此必须对其长期的适用性和维护需求予以充分考虑。

❸ Indirect retainers are supporting elements that act on the opposite end of the axis of rotation of the denture from the saddle to oppose and hinder rotation.
间接固位体作为支撑部件，其位于鞍基在可摘局部义齿转动轴对侧位置的另一端，旨在防止和限制义齿的旋转。

❹ The denture should be reconsidered along with oral hygiene and patient-related factors, such as the patient's manual dexterity to remove and insert the denture.
医生应综合考虑口腔卫生和患者相关因素，如患者取出和佩戴义齿的动手能力，来重新评估和调整可摘局部义齿的设计。

❺ When contemplating prescribing replacement dentures, the clinician should be aware of the basic prosthodontic parameters involved, in addition to assessing the patient's wishes and perceptions.

医生考虑修复方案时，除评估患者的意愿和看法外，还应当掌握相关的基本修复学参数。

⑥ It is essential that the clinician assesses, thoroughly, the denture bearing tissues (DBTs) to determine areas that are unlikely to withstand occlusal loading (e.g., flabby ridges) and which are vulnerable to pressure (e.g., atrophic mucosa, spikey ridges or retained roots).

医生必须对义齿的承托组织进行充分评估，从而确定哪些区域可能无法承受咬合负荷(例如松软的牙槽嵴)，哪些区域容易受压(例如萎缩的黏膜、尖锐的牙槽嵴或残留的牙根)。

⑦ Retention requirements mean that the denture need to create a peripheral seal—essentially a triangle incorporating the post dam as the base and the right and left flanges of the upper denture.

上颌全口义齿的固位需具备良好的边缘封闭——形成一个类三角形，其后部为后堤区，前部为上颌义齿的左右侧翼。

⑧ Finally, the provision of complete dentures does require the harmonious integration of the dental team including the clinician, the dental technician/ clinical dental technician, the dental surgery assistance and the receptionist.

最后，全口义齿的修复离不开精诚合作的团队，包括牙医、技师/椅旁技师、操作助手和接待员。

(本单元由杨宏业选编)

(文字部分选自 *Dentistry at a Glance*, 1st Edition, Part 2, Chapters 55 and 59)

Unit 18 ▸ Extraction of Teeth

1. Introduction

Tooth extraction is a minor surgical procedure and may present with a wide range of difficulty level. Good preoperative assessment and sound extraction technique are essential to achieve a successful outcome with minimal trauma [1]. Straight-forward extractions may be carried out using a closed extraction technique, while more difficult ones may require a surgical approach.

2. Indications

The most common reasons for tooth extraction are unrestorable caries and advanced periodontal disease. Other indications include extensive root resorption (Figure 18.1a), involvement of teeth by pathological lesions (Figure 18.1b), symptomatic impacted and supernumerary teeth (Figure 18.1c), and orthodontic prescriptions. Trauma to teeth and jaw bone may warrant extraction(s). Prophylactic extractions may be required prior to radiotherapy or chemotherapy [2]. Finally, financial constraints may preclude extensive restorative treatment making extraction(s) more feasible option.

3. Contraindications

Local contraindications include a spreading cellulitis and limited mouth opening. However, a localised abscess is not a contraindication as removal of the diseased tooth

---

本单元正文内容选自 Elizabeth Kay 所著 *Dentistry at a Glance*, John Wiley & Sons, Inc., 2016, Chapter 79, pp.166-167, 选用时图片序号有调整。

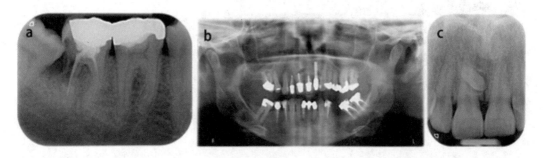

Figure 18.1 （a）Extensive root resorption of a root treated lower right second molar precludes restorative treatment; extraction may be the most appropriate option; （b）A large radicular cyst involving the left mandible molar region; the lesion extends to the lower border of the mandible and failed to resolve following endodontic treatment of the lower left first and second molars; （c）A supernumerary tooth （mesiodens）in the anterior maxilla; this was removed due to persistent discomfort.

（选自 *Dentistry at a Glance*, 1st Edition, Part 2, Chapter 79, Figures 79.1, 79.2 and 79.3）

may offer the most rapid resolution of infection. Nevertheless, obtaining effective local anesthesia may be difficult and this must be considered. Lastly, teeth involved by a malignancy or suspected vascular lesions should not be removed but should be referred for appropriate management.

4.　Preoperative Assessment

4.1　History

Presenting complaints, medical history and patient factors including race, age, and gender.

4.2　Clinical Assessment

Crown form, caries, periodontal health, status and alignment of adjacent teeth, mouth opening.

4.3　Radiographic Assessment

Radiographic assessment may be carried out using a periapical view or an orthpantomogram, or both if appropriate:

    a. Relationship to vital structures (maxillary antrum, inferior alveolar nerve canal, mental foramen).

    b. Root morphology (number, shape, size, curvature).

    c. Evidence of root caries, root resorption, hypercementosis, ankylosis or previous endodontics.

    d. Periradicular pathology (granuoloma, cyst, etc.).

    e. Sclerosis of alveolar bone.

5. Technique

Closed tooth extraction may be carried out using forceps alone but more commonly the tooth is loosened first using an elevator. It is essential that the operator gains adequate access and visualisation of the operative field with correct positioning, use of supporting hand and suction (role of the assistant). An unobstructed path of withdrawal of the tooth must be established and controlled force should be used throughout the extraction [3]. A step-wise approach is as follows:

    a. Detach gingival tissues around the cervical margin of the tooth atraumatically using a periosteal elevator to facilitate application of forceps beaks more apically. This is primarily indicated when extracting a grossly decayed tooth with minimal residual crown.

    b. Loosen the tooth using a luxator and/or a straight elevator.

    c. Adapt the forceps to the tooth and carry out appropriate movements to deliver the tooth (*see* Forceps Extractions).

5.1 Chair and Operator Position

Correct position of the patient, chair and operator is vital during extractions. Ensure that it is comfortable for the operator to approach the tooth, allows adequate visualisation of the field and permits maximal control over force application. Many operators perform extractions in the standing position. For maxillary extractions, the chair is reclined so that the maxillary occlusal plane is 60° to the floor and level with the operator's elbow. For mandibular extractions, the chair is more upright so that the occlusal plane is parallel to the floor and usually 15 cm below the operator's elbow. For all teeth, except mandibular lower right posteriors, the right-handed operator stands in front of the patient on the right side. For mandibular right posteriors, the operator stands behind the patient. These positions are reversed for left-handed operators.

5.2 Role of Non-dominant Hand

a. Reflect the soft tissues (lips, cheeks and tongue) to improve visualisation and minimise trauma.

b. Support the alveolus buccopalatally; this helps to stabilise the patient and gain tactile information to discern tooth movements during extraction.

c. Support the mandible to avoid undue forces being transmitted to the basal bone and temporomandibular joint.

6. Forceps Extractions

Forceps Extraction are used on the wedge principle and facilitate extraction by expanding the socket [4]. After adapting the forceps blades parallel to the long axis of the tooth (Figure 18.2), apical pressure is applied to force the beaks into the gingival sulcus, partially severing the periodontal ligament. Subsequent movements are specific to individual teeth and are summarised below. Slight traction force (pull) is necessary to complete the extraction:

a. Maxillary central incisor (single root): rotation, delivered in a labio-occlusal direction.

b. Maxillary lateral incisor (single root): labial displacement, delivered in a labio-occlusal direction.

c. Maxillary canine (single root): labial force followed by rotation, delivered in a labio-occlusal direction.

d. Maxillary first premolar (two roots): progressive buccopalatal displacement, delivered in an bucco-occlusal direction.

e. Maxillary second premolar (single root): buccal displacement, delivery in bucco-occlusal direction with a rotational traction.

f. Maxillary molars (three roots): progressive buccopalatal displacement, delivery in bucco-occlusal direction.

g. Mandibular incisors and canine (single root): labiolingual displacement followed by rotation, delivery in a labio-occlusal direction.

h. Mandibular premolars (single root): rotation, delivery in bucco-occlusal direction.

i. Mandibular molars (two roots): initially squeeze the beaks into the bifurcation followed by controlled buccal or figure-of-eight movements, delivery in bucco-occlusal direction.

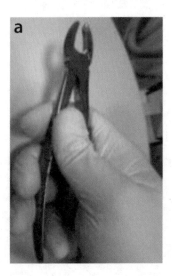 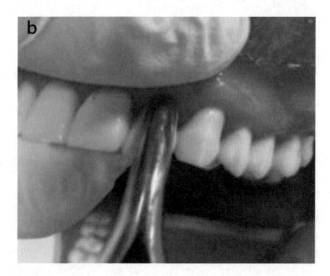

Figure 18.2 (a) Correct way to hold extraction forceps in a palm grip and using little finger to open and close forceps blades; (b) application of forceps on an upper right central incisor with appropriate support of the alveolus using the non-dominant hand.

(选自 *Dentistry at a Glance*, 1st Edition, Part 2, Chapter 79, Figure 79.4)

7. Postextraction Management

Remove any obvious debris such as amalgam, calculus or residual tooth fragments using suction; any residual periapical pathology may be gently curetted. Firmly compress the socket walls using finger pressure buccolingually, taking care not to over-compress if an implant is contemplated. Ensure there are no residual sharp bony projections, which may require smoothening with a bone file [5]. Place a moist gauze pack over the extraction socket for 10 minutes to achieve haemostasis prior to discharging the patient. Written and verbal postextraction instructions should be provided. A review appointment may be arranged for difficult extractions or when complications are likely.

📋 Word List

1. preoperative [prɪˈɒpərətɪv] *adj.* 外科手术前的
2. trauma [ˈtrɔːmə] *n.* 挫折；精神创伤；心理创伤；损伤；外伤
3. orthodontic [ˌɔːθəˈdɒntɪk] *n.* 口腔正畸术；牙齿矫正
4. pathological [ˌpæθəˈlɒdʒɪkl] *adj.* 病理学的；病态的；由疾病引起的
5. symptomatic [ˌsɪmptəˈmætɪk] *adj.* 有症状的；症候的
6. prophylactic [ˌprɒfəˈlæktɪk] *adj.* 预防性的；预防疾病的
7. malignancy [məˈlɪɡnənsi] *n.* 恶性(肿瘤等)；恶意
8. maxillary antrum 上颌窦
9. hypercementosis [ˌhaɪpəsmenˈtəʊsɪs] *n.* 牙骨质增生
10. sclerosis [skləˈrəʊsɪs] *n.* 硬化；硬化症；细胞壁硬化
11. forceps [ˈfɔːseps] *n.* 钳子；医用镊子
12. periosteal [ˌperɪˈɒstɪəl] *adj.* 骨膜的
13. recline [rɪˈklaɪn] *v.* 斜倚
14. maxillary [mækˈsɪləri] *adj.* 上颌骨的；上颌的 *n.* 上颌骨
15. mandibular [mænˈdɪbjʊlə] *adj.* 下颌的；颚的
16. temporomandibular joint (TMJ) 颞下颌关节
17. contemplated [ˈkɒntəmpleɪtɪd] *adj.* 预期的
18. haemostasis [hɪˈmɒstəsɪs] *n.* 止血法

📝 Notes

❶ Good preoperative assessment and sound extraction technique are essential to achieve a successful outcome with minimal trauma.
良好的术前评估和娴熟的拔牙技术是实现微创手术成功的关键。

❷ Prophylactic extractions may be required prior to radiotherapy or chemotherapy.
放疗或化疗前可能需要预防性拔牙。

❸ An unobstructed path of withdrawal of the tooth must be established and controlled force should be used throughout the extraction.
必须建立一个无障碍的拔牙路径，并在整个拔牙过程中使用好控制力。

❹ Forceps extraction are used on the wedge principle and facilitate extraction by expanding the socket.

采用楔的原理，使用拔牙钳扩大牙槽窝以便将牙拔出。

❺ Ensure there are no residual sharp bony projections, which may require smoothening with a bone file.

确保没有残留的尖锐骨突，如果有骨突需要用骨锉进行修整。

（本单元由蔡育选编）

（文字部分选自 *Dentistry at a Glance*, 1st Edition, Part 2, Chapter 79）

Unit 19 ▶ Biopsy

1. Introduction

Biopsy refers to the removal of tissue from a living body for microscopic examination. It is considered the gold standard for diagnosis of pathological lesions and the results of a biopsy dictate the future course of treatment. A systematic approach to diagnosis warrants a detailed medical history, and clinical, radiographic and other relevant investigations. A biopsy helps to establish the true nature of a lesion and may confirm or rule out a malignancy [1]. Biopsies are not routinely performed in general practice; if a dentist has appropriate training and experience, he may carry out biopsies of benign lesions. However, patients with suspected premalignant and malignant lesions must be referred to maxillofacial surgery colleagues. This allows the specialist colleagues to evaluate the patient and helps the formulation of a comprehensive treatment plan without delay.

Indications for a biopsy are:

a. To confirm a clinical diagnosis.

b. To confirm or exclude malignancy.

c. Treatment.

d. May help to monitor progress of a disease.

本单元正文内容选自 Elizabeth Kay 所著 *Dentistry at a Glance*，John Wiley & Sons, Inc., 2016, Chapter 82, pp.172-173，选用时图片序号有改动。

2. Types of Biopsy

2.1　Incisional Biopsy

Incisional biopsy involves removal of only a small portion of a lesion [2]. Generally, a wedge of tissue is removed at the periphery of the lesion to include some normal-appearing tissue in the specimen [3]. It also important to ensure an adequate depth of the tissue by extending the incision margins to the base of a lesion.

Indications for an incisional biopsy are:

a. Suspected premalignant and malignant lesions (Figure 19.1).

b. Large lesions (usually >1 cm).

c. Systemic diseases (e.g. Sjögren syndrome).

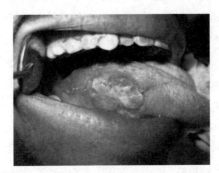

Figure 19.1　A nodular growth on the right lateral border of the tongue in a 23-year-old male; following an incisional biopsy the lesion was diagnosed as a squamous cell carcinoma.

(选自 *Dentistry at a Glance*, 1st Edition, Part 2, Chapter 82, Figure 82.1)

2.2　Excisional Biopsy

Excisional biopsy involves complete removal of the lesion along with a margin of normal tissue (2-3 mm for benign lesions and 4-10 mm for malignant lesions) [4] (Figures 19.2 and 19.3). Generally, a wedge of tissue is removed at the periphery of the lesion to include some normal-appearing tissue in the specimen. Ensure an adequate depth of the tissue by extending the incision margins to the base of a lesion.

Indications for an excisional biopsy are:

163

a. Benign lesions.

b. Small lesions (<1 cm).

Additionally, an excisional biopsy constitutes a definitive treatment by complete removal of the lesion. Common lesions treated by this method include benign fibroepithelial polyp, mucocele and fibroma.

Methods of obtaining a specimen are:

a. Scalpel.

b. Electrocautery.

c. Biopsy forceps/ punch.

d. Lasers.

2.3   Soft Tissue Biopsy

Soft tissue biopsies are mostly carried out using a No.15 surgical blade. Generally, an excisional biopsy of small benign mucosal lesions is performed using an elliptica incisions incorporating 2-3 mm of normal tissue at the periphery [5]. The incisions converge at the base to allow separation of the lesion from underlying connective tissue. Following the removal of a lesion, the wound margins are undermined to facilitate tension-free closure.

Incisional biopsy of large lesions or lesions with suspicion of malignancy (Figure 19.3), is most commonly carried out by outlining a wedge of tissue with a No. 15 surgical scalpel. An alternative is to use a biopsy punch. Essentially the punch comprises a circular blade attached to a plastic handle. Diameters of 2 to 10 mm are available. Multiple incisional biopsies may be required for large lesions with variable surface characteristics [6].

2.4   Bone Biopsy

Intraosseous pathological lesions usually require exposure using a full-thickness mucoperiosteal flap. Care must be observed to avoid damage to important neurovascular structures. Prior to biopsy, aspiration of intraosseous lesions should be done using a 16-18 gauge needle to determine the nature of the lesion (solid or cystic) [7]. The nature of aspirate (fluid, pus, blood, air, etc.) may provide valuable information.

3.   Biopsy Form

A biopsy form provides essential information to the histopathologist to help in

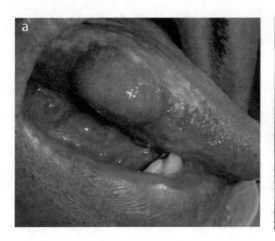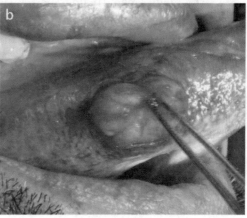

Figure 19.2 （a）A lipoma involving the right lateral border of tongue；（b）Lesion exposed during an excisional biopsy.

Source：Courtesy of Professor MU Akhtar.

（选自 *Dentistry at a Glance*，1st Edition，Part 2，Chapter 82，Figure 82.2）

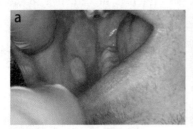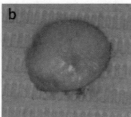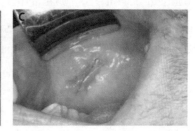

Figure 19.3 （a）A fibroma on the right buccal mucosa；（b）the lesion was excised under local anaesthesia；（c）the surgical site following excision of the lesion and suturing.

（选自 *Dentistry at a Glance*，1st Edition，Part 2，Chapter 82，Figure 82.3）

establishing a correct diagnosis. While the format of the biopsy form may vary，generally the following must be recorded：

    a. Patient's demographic details.

    b. Presenting complaint.

    c. History of presenting complaint.

    d. Past medical and dental history.

    e. Social history.

    f. Clinical description of the lesion（site，size，shape，surface，composition，relationship to nearby structures，status of local tissues，regional lymph nodes，any pertinent systemic findings）.

g. Any radiographic findings (bony lesions).

h. Clinical photographs (soft tissue lesions).

i. Findings of any other investigations.

It is also important to mention the nature of the specimen (soft tissue or bone); the type of biopsy performed (incisional or excisional); any pertinent intraoperative findings and the time-frame for biopsy report (routine or urgent).

4.　Storage and Transport of Specimen

Arrangements for storage and transport of biopsy specimens must be organised before hand by liaising with the histopathology laboratory. For most biopsies, the excised specimen is placed in plastic pot containing a fixative, 10% formalin (4% formaldehyde). Ensure there is an adequate volume of fixative (usually 10 times the volume of the specimen) [8]. The specimen container must also be labelled with patient's and sender's details in case it gets separated from the biopsy form. The specimen is placed in a sealed plastic bag, which should then be placed in a rigid outer container that can be secured by adhesive tape. A further outer padded bag is recommended, which should be labelled 'Pathological specimen' and the name and address of the sender should be clearly displayed.

5.　Adjuncts to Biopsy-cytology

Cytology refers to removal of individual cells for microscopic examination. It is not as reliable as a biopsy and false-negative results are possible. Some applications of cytology for oral pathological lesions include:

a. Oral brush cytology: This technique utilises a hand-held rotator wire brush to collect epithelial cells, which are then fixed on a glass slide for examination. It is mostly used as a tool for screening for oral cancer and monitoring oral precancerous lesions.

b. Fine-needle aspiration cytology: This technique is primarily hospital based. It is used to collect specimens from inaccessible sites, e.g., cervical nodes or salivary glands.

📄 Word List

1. biopsy ['baɪɒpsɪ] *n.* 活组织检查；活组织切片检查；切片检查法
2. comprehensive [ˌkɒmprɪ'hensɪv] *adj.* 综合性的；全面的；有理解力的
3. margin ['mɑːdʒɪn] *n.* 边缘；边际
4. polyp ['pɒlɪp] *n.* 息肉
5. mucocele ['mjuːkəsiːl] *n.* 黏液囊肿
6. elliptical [ɪ'lɪptɪkl] *adj.* 椭圆的
7. intraosseous [ˌɪntrə'ɒsɪəs] *adj.* 骨内的
8. gauge [geɪdʒ] *n.* 口径；直径
9. pertinent ['pɜːtɪnənt] *adj.* 切题的；相关的
10. intraoperative [ˌɪntrə'ɒpərətɪv] *adj.* 手术发生的；术中的
11. adjuncts to biopsy-cytology 辅助活检细胞学检查
12. precancerous [ˌpriː'kænsərəs] *adj.* 癌症前期的
13. nodular ['nɒdjʊlə] *adj.* 结节状的；有结节的
14. lipoma [lɪ'pəʊmə] *n.* 脂肪瘤
15. periphery [pə'rɪfərɪ] *n.* 外围；边缘

✏️ Notes

❶ A biopsy helps to establish the true nature of a lesion and may confirm or rule out a malignancy.
活组织检查有助于确定病变的性质，可以确认或排除恶性肿瘤的可能。

❷ Incisional biopsy involves removal of only a small portion of a lesion.
切取活检只涉及切除病灶的一小部分。

❸ Generally, a wedge of tissue is removed at the periphery of the lesion to include some normal-appearing tissue in the specimen.
通常，活检时在病变的边缘与正常组织交界处切取一块楔状组织。

❹ Excisional biopsy involves complete removal of the lesion along with a margin of normal tissue (2-3 mm for benign lesions and 4-10 mm for malignant lesions).

切除活检包括完全切除病变以及病变周围一定的正常组织(良性病变周围
2~3mm,恶性病变周围4~10mm)。

⑤ Generally, an excisional biopsy of small benign mucosal lesions is performed using
an elliptical incisions incorporating 2-3 mm of normal tissue at the periphery.
一般情况下,对于小的良性黏膜病变,通常使用椭圆形切口进行切除活检,包括
病变周围2~3mm 的正常组织。

⑥ Multiple incisional biopsies may be required for large lesions with variable surface
characteristics.
对于表面特征多样的大型病变,可能需要进行多次切取活检。

⑦ Prior to biopsy, aspiration of intraosseous lesions should be done using a 16-18 gauge
needle to determine the nature of the lesion (solid or cystic).
在活检前,常使用16~18 号针穿刺骨内病变,以确定病变的性质(实性或囊性)。

⑧ Ensure there is an adequate volume of fixative (usually 10 times the volume of the
specimen).
确保有足够量的固定液(通常是标本体积的10 倍)。

(本单元由李瑞芳选编)
(文字部分选自 *Dentistry at a Glance*, 1st Edition, Part 2, Chapter 82)

Unit 20 ▶ Benign Swellings in the Oral Cavity

1. Epithelial Origin

Papilloma is a benign proliferation of stratified squamous epithelium caused by human papilloma virus (HPV). It usually presents as a soft, pedunculated, often exophytic growth. It is painless and the most common sites include the tongue (Figure 20.1a), lips and soft palate. Treatment consists of conservative surgical excision. Recurrence is uncommon.

2. Connective Tissue Origin

2.1 Fibroma

Fibromas are common swellings and represent reactive proliferation of fibrous tissue secondary to local trauma or irritation [1]. They mostly occur on the buccal mucosa along the occlusal line and present as a painless, sessile, smooth-surfaced and firm lump (Figure 20.1b). Treatment consists of conservative surgical excision. Recurrence is rare.

2.2 Pyogenic Granuloma

Pyogenic granuloma is a common benign growth, which results from tissue response

本单元正文内容选自 Elizabeth Kay 所著 *Dentistry at a Glance*, John Wiley & Sons, Inc., 2016, Chapter 286, pp.180-181, 选用时文字内容有少量删减,图片序号有改动。

169

to local irritation or trauma. The term is a misnomer because neither pyogenic organisms are involved nor does it represent a true granuloma. It appears as a soft, highly vascular, pedunculated or sessile lesion. Young adults are most commonly affected with a female predilection. The lesion is painless, tends to bleed and may show rapid growth. If left untreated, most lesions tend to mature with increased collagenisation, which reduces the bleeding. Facial gingival mucosa in the anterior maxilla is the most common site. Involvement of the lips, tongue and buccal mucosa have also been reported. The lesion may develop under the influence of oestrogen and progesterone in pregnant women, hence the terms **pregnancy tumour or granuloma gravidarum** [2]. The histopathological picture is marked by a lobular proliferation of numerous endothelium-lined vascular channels (**lobular capillary haemangioma**) sometimes with ulceration of the surface epithelium. Lesions mature with collagenisation and may present as fibromas. Treatment consists of conservative surgical excision. In pregnant women, treatment may be delayed until parturition to allow spontaneous regression; otherwise the recurrence rate may be high.

2.3   Denture Hyperplasia

Inflammatory, reactive proliferation of fibrous connective tissue may present in several forms in association with ill-fitting dentures:

a. **Epulis fissuratum** : Develops on the alveolar vestibule as multiple folds of hyperplastic tissue bordering a denture flange, usully in the anterior region (Figure 20.1c).

b. **Leaf-like denture fibroma or fibroepithelial polyp** : It appears as a pedunculated mass of fibrous tissue attached to the palate.

c. **Papillary hyperplasia (denture papillomatosis)**: Develops on the palate underneath a maxillary denture and appears as a papillary and erythematous lesion (Figure 20.2a). Candida may possibly be involved.

Treatment consists of surgical excision and correction or replacement of ill-fitting denture. Denture papillomatosis may respond to discontinuation of denture use and antifungal therapy in early stages [3].

2.4   Gingival Fibromatosis

Gingival fibromatosis is characterized by proliferation of fibrous connective tissue and

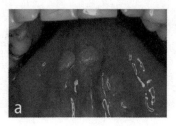 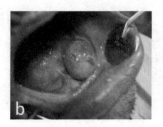 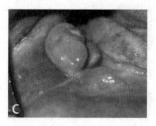

Figure 20.1   (a) Ventral aspect of the tongue showing two discrete sessile papillomas. Source: Courtesy of Professor Mao Lewis; (b) Clinical photograph of a large fibroma involving the left mandibular alveolar ridge in an edentulous subject; (c) An epulis fissuratum on the lower edentulous ridge; note the groove on the surface of the lesion to accommodate the denture flange.

(选自 *Dentistry at a Glance*, 1st Edition, Part 2, Chapter 86, Figure 86.1, Figure 86.2 and Figure 86.3)

may be localised or generalised. Although more common in children and adolescents, the condition may be observed in adults (Figure 20.2b). Treatment usually requires surgical excision of the lesional tissue.

2.5   Peripheral Giant Cell Granuloma

Peripheral giant cell granuloma is a benign reactive proliferation secondary to local irritation or trauma and may represent a soft tissue counterpart of central giant cell granuloma. It presents as a reddish blue mass on the gingivae or edentulous alveolar mucosa (Figure 20.2c). It is usually seen in the fifth and sixth decades with a female predilection. The histopathological picture is characterised by the presence of multinucleated giant cells. Treatment consists of surgical excision.

2.6   Lipoma

Lipomas are benign lumps of fatty tissue and are uncommon in the oral cavity. They present a soft, lobulated painless lump, usually involving the buccal mucosa (Figure 20.2d). They are usually identified in mature adults, and there is no gender predilection. The histopathological picture is marked by proliferation of mature fatcells. Treatment consists of conservative surgical excision.

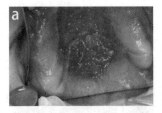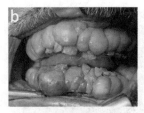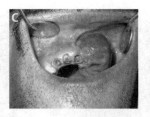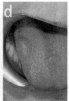

Figure 20.2 （a）Papillary hyperplasia of the palate in a patient with a poorly fitting upper full denture；（b）Remarkable untreated generalized gingival fibromatosis in an adult male. （c）A peripheral giant cell granuloma involving the left maxilla；（d）A lipoma involving the right lateral border of tongue.

Source：Figure(b) and (d), courtesy of Professor MU Akhtar.

（选自 *Dentistry at a Glance*, 1st Edition, Part 2, Chapter 86,Figures 86.4, 86.5, 86.6 and 86.7）

3. Vascular Origin

3.1 Haemangioma

Haemangioma is a benign hamartomatous proliferation of endothelial cells in infants ［4］. It is most commonly observed in the first year of life, displaying rapid growth in the first few months and is more common in females. Most lesions are confined to soft tissues and are well circumscribed. Superficial lesions are usually bright red, while deeper lesions may have a bluish hue. Most lesions regress spontaneously by the fifth year and do not require any treatment.

3.2 Vascular Malformations

Vascular malformations represent abnormalities of vessel morphogenesis without endothelial proliferation ［5］. They are present at birth and tend to persist throughout life （Figures 20.3a）. They may involve the soft tissues or bone and are classified on the basis of type of vessel involved （capillary, arterial, venous） and flow rate （low flow or high flow）. A **port wine stain** represents a capillary malformation, which may appear as a pink or purple lesion in the distribution of the trigeminal nerve ［6］ （Figures 20.3b and 20.3c）. Venous malformations are low-flow lesions while arteriovenous malformations are typically high-flow lesions with an audible bruit or thrill. Vascular malformations involving the bone may present with bony expansion and often appear as a multilocular radiolucent defect. Treatment options include sclerotherapy or therapeutic embolization followed by surgical resection. It is wise to perform needle aspiration on an undiagnosed bony pathology in the jaws to rule out a vascular malformation prior to extractions or surgery.

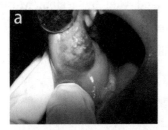 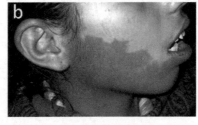 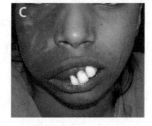

Figure 20.3 (a) A large soft tissue vascular malformation involving the left buccal mucosa in a 14-year old female; (b) An extensive port wine stain involving the right lower face and neck; (c) A port wine stain involving the right mid-face. The patient also had a large vascular malformation of the right maxilla. Source: Figure(c), courtesy of Professor MU Akhtar.

(选自 *Dentistry at a Glance*, 1st Edition, Part 2, Chapter 86, Figures 86.8, 86.9 and 86.10)

3.3 Lymphangioma

Lymphangioma is a benign, hamartomatous proliferation of lymphatic vessels and presents in the first few years [7]. The anterior part of the tongue is the most common site for oral lesions. Treatment consists of surgical excision, although complete removal may be difficult. The recurrence rate is generally high.

4. Neural 'Lumps'

4.1 Neurofibroma

Neurofibroma is a benign lump, which develops from Schwaan cells and perineural fibroblasts. It is the most common peripheral nerve tumour and typically occurs in young adults. It presents as a slow-growing, soft, painless lump on the skin, tongue or buccal mucosa. Treatment consists of conservative surgical excision and recurrence is rare. Multiple neurofibromas may develop due to a hereditary disease, neurofibromatosis (von Recklinghausen disease).

4.2   Traumatic Neuroma

Traumatic neuroma is a benign, reactive proliferation of neural tissue at the site of nerve damage due to trauma or surgery. Pain may be associated with the lesion. Most develop in the region of the mental foramen but may also be seen on the tongue and lower lip. Treatment consists of conservative surgical excision. Recurrence is rare.

📄 **Word List**

1. papilloma [ˌpæpɪˈləʊmə] *n.* 乳头状瘤
2. exophytic [ˈeksəfaɪtɪk] *adj.* 外部生长的
3. pyogenic granuloma 化脓性肉芽肿
4. oestrogen [ˈiːstrədʒən] *n.* 雌激素
5. erythematous [ˌerɪˈθiːmətəs] *adj.* 红斑的
6. edentulous [iːˈdentʃələs] *adj.* 缺齿的；无齿的
7. lobulated [ˈlɒbjʊleɪtɪd] *adj.* 分成小叶的
8. predilection [ˌpriːdɪˈlekʃn] *n.* 偏爱；嗜好
9. haemangioma [ˌhɪmændʒɪˈəʊmə] *n.* 血管瘤
10. spontaneously [spɒnˈteɪnɪəslɪ] *adv.* 自发地；不由自主地；自然地
11. vascular malformation 脉管畸形
12. morphogenesis [ˌmɔːfəˈdʒenɪsɪs] *n.* 形态发生
13. trigeminal [traɪˈdʒemɪnl] *adj.* 三叉神经的
14. bruit [bruːt] *n.* (尤指听诊中听到的)杂音
15. multilocular [ˌmʌltɪˈlɒkjʊlə] *adj.* 多室的；多腔的
16. lymphangioma [lɪmˌfændʒɪˈəʊmə] *n.* 淋巴管瘤
17. hamartomatous proliferation of lymphatic vessels 淋巴管错构瘤增生
18. neurofibroma [ˌnjʊərəʊfaɪˈbrəʊmə] *n.* 神经纤维瘤
19. traumatic neuroma 创伤性神经瘤

✎ Notes

① Fibromas are common swellings and represent reactive proliferation of fibrous tissue secondary to local trauma or irritation.
纤维瘤是常见的肿块，是纤维组织受到局部创伤或刺激后的反应性增生。

② The lesion may develop under the influence of oestrogen and progesterone in pregnant women, hence the terms pregnancy tumour or granuloma gravidarum.
该病变（化脓性肉芽肿）可在孕妇体内雌激素和黄体酮的影响下发生，因此称为妊娠期肿瘤或妊娠性肉芽肿。

③ Denture papillomatosis may respond to discontinuation of denture use and antifungal therapy in early stages.
义齿相关乳头瘤病可能在早期阶段停止使用义齿和进行抗真菌治疗后有所缓解。

④ Haemangioma is a benign hamartomatous proliferation of endothelial cells in infants.
血管瘤是一种婴儿内皮细胞良性错构瘤性增殖形成的病变。

⑤ Vascular malformations represent abnormalities of vessel morphogenesis without endothelial proliferation.
血管畸形表现为血管形态发生异常，无内皮细胞增殖。

⑥ A port wine stain represents a capillary malformation, which may appear as a pink or purple lesion in the distribution of the trigeminal nerve.
葡萄酒色斑是毛细血管畸形的一种，可表现为三叉神经分布区域内的粉红或紫色病变。

⑦ Lymphangioma is a benign, hamartomatous proliferation of lymphatic vessels and presents in the first few years.
淋巴管瘤是一种良性的错构瘤样淋巴管增生，通常发生于生命的最初几年。

（本单元由尚政军选编）
（文字部分选自 *Dentistry at a Glance*, 1st Edition, Part 2, Chapter 86）

Unit 21 ▶ Odontogenic Tumours and Tumour-like Lesions

1. Introduction

Odontogenic tumours develop from odontogenic epithelium, odontogenic ectomesenchyme or both (mixed) and are classified accordingly. They display varied clinical and histopathologica features, and treatments are different for each type of tumour.

2. Tumours of Odontogenic Epithelium

2.1 Ameloblastoma

Ameloblastoma is the most common odontogenic tumour excluding odontomas. It may originate from a variety of epithelial tissues, including the dental lamina, enamel organ, or sometimes from the lining of an odontogenic cyst [1]. It is a slow-growing, locally aggressive neoplasm and may present with several distinct clinical radiographic appearances (Figure 21.1).

The **solid or multicystic** variety is the most common type and is usually seen in adult patients over a wide age range without any gender predilection. The posterior of the mandible is the most common site and the ameloblastoma usually presents as a painless expansion of the jaws [2]. Radiographically, the multicystic type presents as a multilocular radiolucency, simulating either a 'soap bubble' or 'honey comb' appearance.

本单元正文内容选自 Elizabeth Kay 所著 *Dentistry at a Glance*, John Wiley & Sons, Inc., 2016, Chapter 87, pp.182-183, 选用时图片序号有改动。

Buccal cortical expansion and root resorption of adjacent teeth may be seen. The solid variety appears as a unilocular radiolucency.

The histopathological picture is varied, with the **follicular** pattern being the most common [3]. It is characterised by islands of enamel organ-type epithelium with reversed polarity. The epithelium encloses a core of loose, stellate reticulum-type cells and is surrounded by a fibrous connective tissue. Areas of cystic degeneration are common. The **plexiform** pattern displays cords or sheets of odontogenic epithelium enclosing loosely arranged epithelium and a loose, vascular connective tissue. Other patterns include: **acanthomatous** (epithelium with squamous metaplasia and keratin formation); granular cell (epithelium displays eosinophilic granules); **desmoplastic** (a dense collagen stroma); or **basal cell** (cuboidal epithelial cells).

Multicystic or solid ameloblastoma is an aggressive tumour with a high recurrence rate [4]. Treatment options range from enucleation to enblocresection. However, marginal resection with a 1-cm border past the radiographic limits of the lesion is recommended.

Unicystic and **peripheral** variants are also seen (Figure 21.2). They respond to enucleation or conservative excision.

2.2 Malignant Ameloblastoma and Ameloblastic Carcinoma

Rarely, an ameloblastoma may develop malignant changes and show metastases [5]. **Malignant ameloblastoma** shows histopathological features of ameloblastoma, both in the primary as well as metastatic lesions. Ameloblastic carcinoma shows histopathological features of malignancy in a primary, recurrent or metastatic lesion [6].

2.3 Adenomatoid Odontogenic Tumour

These tumours develop from the epithelium of enamel organ or dental lamina and are mainly seen in younger patients (10-19 years) with a female predilection. The anterior part of the maxilla is the most common site and it usually presents as an asymptomatic lesion. It may cause delayed eruption of involved teeth, prompting radiographic investigations (Figure 21.3). Radiographically, it presents as a well-circumscribed radiolucency, often with scattered foci of calcification. The histopathological picture is marked by tubular epithelial structures simulating preameloblasts with a central space, foci

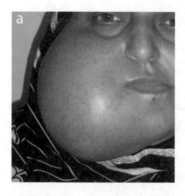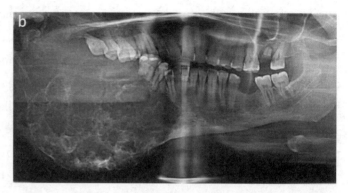

Figure 21.1   Clinical（a）and radiographic view（b）of a grotesque ameloblastoma involving the right mandible in a 40-year old female. The lesion has a classical multilocular radiographic appearance with evidence of root resorption of adjacent teeth.

Source：Courtesy of Professor MU Akhtar.

（选自 *Dentistry at a Glance*，1st Edition，Part 2，Chapter 87，Figure 87.1）

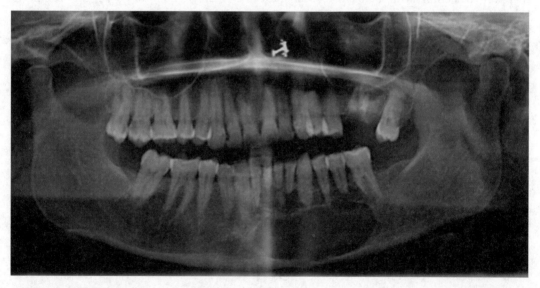

Figure 21.2   OPG of a unicystic ameloblastoma involving the left mandible in a 38-year-old female；note root resorption of adjacent teeth.

Source：Courtesy of Professor MU Akhtar.

（选自 *Dentistry at a Glance*，1st Edition，Part 2，Chapter 87，Figure 87.2）

of calcification（dentinoid or cementum）and a fibrous capsule. Treatment involves a conservative enucleation. Peripheral variants are reported.

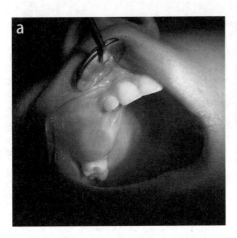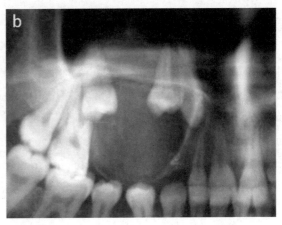

Figure 21.3   Clinical (a) and radiographic view (b) of an adenomatoid odontogenic tumour involving the right maxilla in a 13-year-old female child; the lesion has prevented the eruption of multiple teeth.

(选自 *Dentistry at a Glance*, 1st Edition, Part 2, Chapter 87, Figure 87.3)

2.4   Calcifying Epithelial Odontogenic Tumour

Also known as **Pindborg** tumour, this develops from the epithetlium of dental lamina. It is an uncommon lesion and is mainly seen in mature adults with no gender predilection. The posterior of the mandible is the most common site and it usually presents as a painless swelling. Radiographically, it presents as a multilocular or unilocular radiolucency interspersed with varying amounts of calcified structures. Histopathological picture is marked by islands of polyhedral epithelial cells with a fibrous stroma. Large areas of eosinophilic, amyloid-like material may be present extracellularly and display foci of calcification. Treament involves a marginal resection with a narrow rim of normal bone. Peripheral variants are reported.

Other odontogenic tumours of epithelial origin include squamous odontogenic tumour and clear-cell odontogenic carcinoma [7].

3. Mixed Odontogenic Tumours

This group includes odontomas, ameloblastic fibroma, ameloblastic fibro-odontoma, ameloblastic sarcoma, odontoamelo blastoma and odontomes.

3.1 Odontoma

Odontomas constitute the most common type of odontogenic tumours and are better termed dental hamartomas [8]. They develop from odontogenic epithelium and mesenchyme, resulting in formation of dental tissues. They are usually asymptomatic but may prevent tooth eruption in the involved area. Most are discovered following dental radiographs to investigate missing teeth. **Compound odontomas** are composed of multiple small tooth-like structures and tend to involve the anterior maxilla. **Complex odontomas** appear as a radiopaque mass of disorganised dental tissue and are more common in the posterior area of the jaws. Odontomas are treated by conservative surgical removal.

3.2 Ameloblastic Fibroma

Ameloblastic fibroma is an uncommon lesion and is mainly seen during the first two decades of life. The posterior part of the mandible is the most common site and it is usually asymptomatic. Radiographically, it presents as a well-defined unilocular or multilocular radiolucency. Small lesions can be treated with curettage but marginal resection is warranted for recurrences.

4. Tumours of Odontogenic Mesenchyme

This group includes odontogenic fibroma, granular cell odontogenic tumour, odontogenic myxoma and cementoblastoma.

4.1 Odontogenic Myxoma

Odontogenic myxoma develops from odontogenic mesenchyme and is mainly seen in young adults (20-30 years) with no gender predilection [9]. The posterior of the mandible is the most common site and it is usually asymptomatic or presents as a painless jaw expansion. Radiographically, it presents as a unilocular or multilocular radiolucency and may cause root resorption of adjacent teeth. Histopathological features include spindle-shaped or round cells in a loose, myxoid stroma. Myxomas may be treated with curettage but recurrence warrants marginal resection.

4.2   Cementoblastoma

Cementoblastoma is uncommon but is the only true neoplasm of cementum (Figure 21.4). It is mainly identified in children and young adults with no gender predilection. The posterior mandible is the most common site and the tumour classically involves the lower first permanent molar. It may present with jaw swelling and pain but can also be asymptomatic. Radiographically, it presents as a radiopaque mass attached to the root of an involved tooth. The histopathological picture simulates an osteoblastoma and is marked by mineralised deposits with irregular lacunae and prominent basophilic reversal lines. Treatment options include surgical removal of the calcified mass combined with either extraction or root amputation (after endodontics) of the involved tooth.

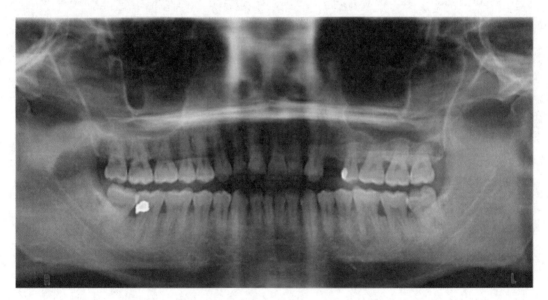

Figure 21.4   A well-demarcated mixed radiopaque and radiolucent lesion associated with the mesial root of LL6; the tooth is free from caries or periodontal disease and is vital. The lesion was diagnosed as a cementoblastoma. Note the mental foramen just below the lesion.

(选自 *Dentistry at a Glance*, 1st Edition, Part 2, Chapter 87, Figure 87.4)

📄 Word List

1. ameloblastoma [ˌæməlɒblæsˈtəmə] n. 成釉细胞瘤；造釉细胞瘤；釉母细胞瘤
2. neoplasm [ˈniː(ː)əʊplæzm] n. 赘生物；瘤；新生物
3. cortical [ˈkɔːtɪkəl] adj. 皮质的；皮层的；外皮的
4. unilocular [ˌjuːnɪˈlɒkjʊlə] adj. 单室的；单房的
5. follicular [fəˈlɪkjʊlə] adj. 滤泡的；卵泡的；小囊的
6. stellate [ˈsteˌleɪt] adj. 星形的；似星的；放射线状的
7. plexiform [ˈpleksɪfɔːm] adj. (血管等)丛状的
8. desmoplastic [dezˈmɒplæstɪk] adj. 促结缔组织增生的
9. asymptomatic [ˌeɪsɪmptəˈmætɪk] adj. 无症状的
10. calcification [ˌkælsɪfɪˈkeɪʃn] n. 钙化；石灰化
11. polyhedral [ˌpɒlɪˈhiːdrəl] adj. 多面的；多面体的
12. eosinophilic [ˌiːə'sɪnəˈfɪlɪk] adj. 嗜酸性的
13. odontoma [ɒdɒnˈtəmə] n. 牙瘤
14. hamartomas [ˌhæmɑːˈtəʊmə] n. 错构瘤
15. mesenchyme [ˈmezənkaɪm] n. 间质
16. ameloblastic fibroma 成釉细胞纤维瘤

✏️ Notes

❶ It may originate from a variety of epithelial tissues, including the dental lamina, enamel organ, or sometimes from the lining of an odontogenic cyst.
它可能来源于多种上皮组织，包括牙板、成釉器，或牙源性囊肿的衬里上皮。

❷ The posterior of the mandible is the most common site and the ameloblastoma usually presents as a painless expansion of the jaws.
成釉细胞瘤最常见的好发部位是下颌骨后部，通常表现为颌骨的无痛性膨隆。

❸ The histopathological picture is varied, with the follicular pattern being the most common.
(成釉细胞瘤的)组织病理学表现多种多样，其中滤泡型最为常见。

❹ Multicystic or solid ameloblastoma is an aggressive tumour with a high recurrence rate.
多囊型或实性型成釉细胞瘤是一种高复发率的侵袭性肿瘤。

❺ Rarely, an ameloblastoma may develop malignant changes and show metastases.
极少情况下，成釉细胞瘤可能发生恶变，并出现转移。

❻ Ameloblastic carcinoma shows histopathological features of malignancy in a primary, recurrent or metastatic lesion.
成釉细胞癌是指表现出恶性组织病理学特征的原发性、复发性或转移性成釉细胞瘤。

❼ Other odontogenic tumours of epithelial origin include squamous odontogenic tumour and clear-cell odontogenic carcinoma.
其他上皮来源的牙源性肿瘤包括牙源性鳞状细胞瘤和牙源性透明细胞癌。

❽ Odontomas constitute the most common type of odontogenic tumours and are better termed dental hamartomas.
牙瘤是最常见的牙源性肿瘤，更确切地说，牙瘤是牙错构瘤。

❾ Odontogenic myxoma develops from odontogenic mesenchyme and is mainly seen in young adults (20-30 years) with no gender predilection.
牙源性黏液瘤由牙源性间充质发展而来，主要见于 20~30 岁的年轻成人，无性别偏好。

（本单元由陈刚选编）
（文字部分选自 *Dentistry at a Glance*，1st Edition，Part 2，Chapter 87）

Unit 22 ▶ Implant-retained Options

1. Indications for Implant-retained Prostheses

Replacement of missing teeth can be challenging, as bone is lost both immediately and gradually following tooth loss. Implants provide a means by which a prosthesis can be attached directly to bone without the involvement of adjacent teeth. A successful outcome for this treatment is contingent upon the prognosis for the surrounding dentition, the presence of favourable healing conditions to facilitate osseointegration and favourable bone volume [1]. There are very few absolute contraindications to implant surgery, but any factor that compromises good healing is a relative contraindication. This would include poorly controlled diabetes mellitus and prolonged use of bisphosphonate medication (particularly IV bisphosphonates). Smoking is not a contraindication per se, but cigarette smoking adversely influences treatment outcomes.

When anterior teeth are missing, particularly those in the aesthetic zone, it is vital that the clinician fully understands the patient's expectations for treatment in advance of placing dental implants. It is important to remember that a prosthesis is required to replace teeth and associated bone, and this is not always straightforward when a fixed prosthesis is planned. On the other hand, a removable partial denture (RPD), by virtue of having teeth and a flange, presents a means of replacing lost teeth and bone more readily. In an ideal world, teeth would be replaced as soon as they were lost. However, this is highly unusual and the longer the delay in replacing teeth with implant-retained restorations, the more complex the replacement challenge becomes. Ideally, implants would be placed within 8 weeks of tooth loss. Where there is congenital absence of permanent teeth, the

本单元正文内容选自 Elizabeth Kay 所著 *Dentistry at a Glance*, John Wiley & Sons, Inc., 2016, Chapter 54, pp.114-115, 选用时图片序号有改动。

alveolar ridge in the area of absent teeth is very narrow. In these situations, the alveolar ridge has to be augmented prior to placing implants (Figure 22.1a) or at the time of implant placement (Figure 22.1b). A further consideration is the condition of the soft tissues at the implant site and the gingival biotype. If the patient has a thin biotype with a high smile line, it is very challenging. A thick tissue biotype with a low smile line is far less problematic (Figure 22.1c).

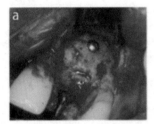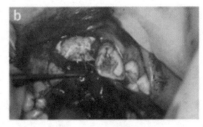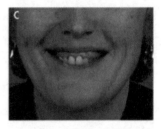

Figure 22.1　(a) Reduced bone volume, augmented with an onlay bone graft; (b) Exposed implant threads covered with autogenous bone chips and a membrane; (c) High smile line, which would present complex aesthetic management problems.

（选自 *Dentistry at a Glance*, 1st edition, Part 2, Chapter 54, Figures 54.1, 54.2 and 54.3)

The specific indications for implant-retained prostheses in partially dentate patients include:

a. A healthy dentition where teeth have been lost to trauma (Figures 22.2a and 22.2b).

b. Missing teeth with unrestored teeth adjacent to the space.

c. Diastema present in the area where the tooth has been lost (Figure 22.2c).

d. Unfavourable span for conventional fixed prosthodontics.

e. Patients with congenital absence of teeth (Figure 22.2d).

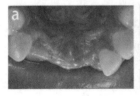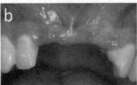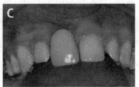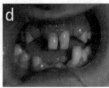

Figure 22.2　(a, b) Maxillary anterior teeth lost to trauma, long span, surrounding dentition unrestored: (a) Occlusal view; (b) Labial view; (c) Diastema adjacent to missing tooth currently restored with an RPD; note also the significant soft and hard tissue deficit causing poor appearance; (d) Patient with congenital absence of teeth (hypodontia); note narrow alveolar ridge in area of missing teeth.

（选自 *Dentistry at a Glance*, 1st Edition, Part 2, Chapter 54, Figures 54.4, 54.5 and 54.6)

2.　Planning Procedures

When planning tooth replacement, it is important to ensure that pathology and unfavourable occlusal forces are controlled. If the patient exhibits signs of parafunction, this can cause delayed failure of implants. It is also important to ensure that heavy excursive forces are not introduced into an implant-retained crown or bridge restoration. Further examination requirements include:

a. Assessment of alveolar bone width and height (clinical and radiographic examination).

b. Mesiodistal distance between teeth.

c. Interocclusal space assessment (particularly relevant posteriorly).

d. Assessment of soft tissues and presence or absence of papilla.

e. Height of smile line (very high lip line is challenging).

Aids to planning include the use of plain film radiographs and good-quality mounted study casts. Three-dimensional imaging is advisable when teeth are lost either due to trauma or chronic infection, as significant bone volume deficit is likely in these cases.

The positioning and placement of implants must be related to the desired cosmetic outcome. A diagnostic wax-up cast is essential to help simulate the appearance of the final restoration and evaluate whether it is acceptable to the patient [2]. The wax-up can be based on a previously satisfactory restoration (e.g., a failed conventional bridge or RPD). Alternatively, it can be done de novo and altered until the patient is satisfied (Figure 22.3a). In addition to establishing what the patient expects in terms of appearance, the wax-up can also help determine if sufficient tissue is available to achieve this appearance at the end of treatment. In conjunction with the radiographic information, the need for bony ridge augmentation and connective tissue grafting can be decided.

The final wax-up is then used to fabricate a surgical stent to guide implant placement (Figure 22.3b). It is essential that the operator placing the implants uses the surgical guide to ensure optimal placement.

3.　Surgical Phase

A standardised protocol is use to place implants, and it is important that there is careful handling of soft and hard tissues. Good irrigation is essential, and controlled drill

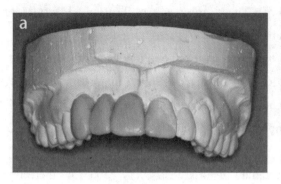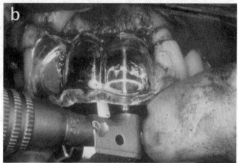

Figure 22.3 (a) Diagnostic wax-up cast; (b) Surgical stent based on diagnostic wax-up used to guide placement of implant.

(选自 *Dentistry at a Glance*, 1st Edition, Part 2, Chapter 54, Figures 54.7, 54.8)

speed is used to avoid damaging bone. With the aid of the surgical stent, pilot holes are used to check the orientation of the implant site as it is being prepared. Any granulation tissue or foreign body material in the implant site should be completely debrided.

The implant site should be gradually widened to the predetermined length and diameter, and the implant itself then placed. It is important to get good primary stability of the implant in the bone [3]. Where implant threads are exposed, these should be covered with an autogenous bone graft material with a membrane to facilitate bone regeneration over the exposed threads. Depending on the stability of the implant, it can then be covered with a healing cap and the mucoperiosteal flap sutured around this, or covered with the flap for a period of 4-6 months to facilitate osseointegration.

4. Restorative Phase

Once initial healing has occurred, the restorative treatment can commence. Implants have successfully osseointegrated when there a torque force exerted on the implant elicits neither movement nor pain. The normal treatment sequence is as follows:

a. Primary impression, followed by a 'pick-up' impression in a customised impression tray using premachined impression copings. An interocclusal record should be sent with this and an opposing cast to the laboratory.

b. Once cast, either premachined or customised transmucosal abutment components are used to retain the crown or bridge-work (Figures 22.4a and 22.4b). In the aesthetic zone, use of provisional restorations to shape soft tissues is recommended [4] (Figure 22.4c). These are made of heat-cured acrylic or composite resin materials, which are easy to adjust as required.

c. Once the final shape of soft tissues has been achieved and any occlusal adjustments have been made, the final restoration can be made. A new impression is made, and the crown or bridge is fabricated. This can be cement or screw retained, depending on the position of the implant and the need for retrievability (Figure 22. 4).

The long-term prognosis for implant-retained restorations is very good, but there is a degree of maintenance required [5]. It is important that the patient maintains a good standard of oral hygiene to avoid peri-implant soft tissue inflammation.

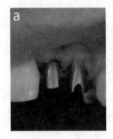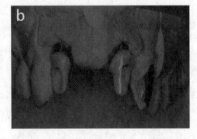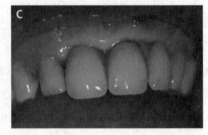

Figure 22.4　Customised abutments connected to implants: (a) Titanium; (b) Zirconia; (c) Provisional restoration used to shape the papillae postsurgery; note blanching of tissues around restorations.

(选自 *Dentistry at a Glance*, 1st Edition, Part 2, Chapter 54, Figures 54.9, 54.10)

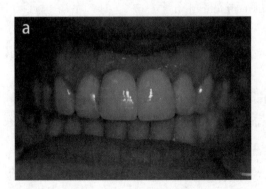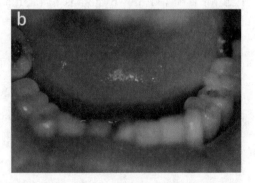

Figure 22.5　(a) Cement-retained restoration replacing maxillary central incisors; (b) screw-retained restoration replacing lower left second premolar.

(选自 *Dentistry at a Glance*, 1st Edition, Part 2, Chapter 54, Figure 54.11)

📋 Word List

1. implant [ɪmˈplɑːnt] *n.* 种植体
2. osseointegration [ˌɒsiːəʊɪntɪɡˈreɪʃn] *n.* 骨整合
3. wax-up [ˈwæks-ʌp] *n.* 蜡型
4. surgical stent 手术导板
5. primary stability 初期稳定性
6. healing cap 愈合基台
7. impression [ɪmˈpreʃən] *n.* 印模
8. abutment [əˈbʌtmənt] *n.* 基台
9. provisional restorations 临时修复体
10. cement-retained [sɪˈment-rɪˈteɪnd] *adj.* 粘接固位
11. screw-retained [skruː-rɪˈteɪnd] *adj.* 螺丝固位
12. maintenance [ˈmeɪntənəns] *n.* (种植体周)维护

✍ Notes

❶ A successful outcome for this treatment is contingent upon the prognosis for the surrounding dentition, the presence of favourable healing conditions to facilitate osseointegration and favourable bone volume.
种植治疗的成功取决于邻牙的预后、有利于骨整合的愈合条件，以及充足的骨量。

❷ The positioning and placement of implants must be related to the desired cosmetic outcome. A diagnostic wax-up cast is essential to help simulate the appearance of the final restoration and evaluate whether it is acceptable to the patient.
种植体的植入位置与理想的美学修复效果息息相关，因此有必要制作诊断蜡型来模拟最终修复体的外观，从而评估患者是否接受最终修复效果。

❸ The implant site should be gradually widened to the predetermined length and diameter, and the implant itself then placed. It is important to get good primary stability of the implant in the bone.

种植位点应当逐级预备达到理想的长度和直径，然后植入种植体。种植体在骨内获得良好的初期稳定性是十分重要的。

❹　In the aesthetic zone, use of provisional restorations to shape soft tissues is recommended.

在美学区，推荐使用临时修复体进行种植体牙龈软组织塑形。

❺　The long-term prognosis for implant-retained restorations is very good, but there is a degree of maintenance required.

尽管种植体支持式义齿的长期修复效果良好，但仍离不开一定程度的后期维护。

（本单元由张玉峰选编）

（文字部分选自 *Dentistry at a Glance*, 1st Edition, Part 2, Chapter 54）

Unit 23 ▶ Reading and Reporting Radiographs

1. Reading Radiographs

There are many necessary requirements for adequately reading and interpreting dental radiographs and some of these include:

1.1 Optimal Viewing Conditions

For traditional radiographs, the requirements are a dry radiograph, an even, uniform, bright light viewing screen (Figure 23.1), a dark surround around the radiograph so that light only passes through the film and the use of a magnifying glass. For digital systems the requirements to view the radiograph are: optimal contrast, brightness and image enhancement, and use of a zoom facility [1].

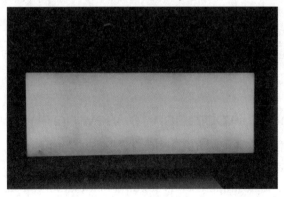

Figure 23.1   A traditional X-ray viewer.

本单元正文内容选自 Elizabeth Kay 所著 *Dentistry at a Glance*, John Wiley & Sons, Inc., 2016, Chapter 12, pp.24-25, 选用时已删除原文所有图片, 本单元图片为本单元作者提供; 另外选用时文字内容有改动。

1.2 Knowledge of the Radiographic Appearance of Normal Anatomical Structures

It is especially important to be able to differentiate between healthy teeth, normal periodontal tissues and other normal structures such as foramina, bone trabeculae, the inferior dental nerve canal, etc., and pathological features.

1.3 Knowledge of the Radiographic Appearance of Pathology That May Affect the Dental Region

It is important to recognize dental caries and periodontal disease on radiographs but also necessary to be able to recognise less common pathology such as cysts and tumours etc.

1.4 Knowledge and Understanding of What Dental Radiographs Should Look Like

This is so that quality assurance and reporting can be carried out accurately.

1.5 Access to Previous Radiographs So That Comparisons Can Be Made

This is important so that key features and the progression of lesions can be ascertained, e.g., caries, apical pathology, bone loss and the rate of development can be measured.

1.6 A Systematic Approach to Viewing the Entire Radiograph and Pathology-specific Areas

A systematic and logical approach is so important that all relevant information is read and reported correctly. Suggestions for a systematic sequence for reporting radiographs should include:

a. Teeth

Record missing teeth

Record the findings relevant to the crowns of the teeth: caries/restorations, etc.

Record the findings relevant to the roots of the teeth: fillings, resorption, length, fractures, caries, etc.

Record the findings of the apices: nothing abnormal detected, radiolucencies, opacities, obturation material, etc.

b. Periodontal tissues

Record any calculus deposits

Record bone loss, vertical and horizontal

Note furcation involvement

Record any widening of the periodontal ligament

With dental panoramic tomographic (DPT) radiographs note the mandible shape, thickness, condyle anatomy, foramina, border, trabeculae, antra, etc.

c. Pathology: a description of a pathological lesion should include:

Location of the lesion, e.g., apex, crown, interdental, mesial, distal, horizontal, vertical, anterior, posterior, within an antrum, etc.

Size of the lesion, give a measurement in mm, e.g., 5 mm in diameter.

Shape and nature of the lesion, e.g., oval, round, regular, irregular, radiopaque, radiolucent, etc.

Proximity to other structures when comparing to previous radiographs, try to ascertain the time that lesion has been present.

2. Reporting Radiographs

Justification for the radiograph should always be recorded in the patient's notes, for example caries screen, bone levels, apical pathology, etc. Radiographs should be labelled correctly (traditional films) with the name of the patient, date radiograph was taken, dentist who prescribed the radiograph and identification of the tooth that was X-rayed (e.g., Joe Bloggs, PA of LR7, 23rd October 2012 and initials of dentist).

The findings from the systematic and logical examination of the radiograph, including teeth, periodontal structures and pathology, should be documented in the patient's notes.

3. Quality Assurance

Being able to report on radiographs is imperative to maintaining good quality and high standards of dental care. The World Health Organisation (WHO) has defined radiographic quality assurance (QA) programmes as 'an organized effort by the staff operating a facility to ensure that the diagnostic images produced by the facility are of sufficiently high quality so that they consistently provide adequate diagnostic information at the lowest possible cost and with the least possible exposure of the patient to radiation' [2]. Rating a radiograph falls into one of three categories.

- Quality assurance 1 (QA1) Excellent—no errors. Patient positioning is correct as well as the film being positioned correctly. Exposure time should be correct for size of patient and position of the tooth/ teeth with no processing or handling faults [3]. QA1 (Excellent) being the optimal score and when auditing radiographs should be no less than 70% of all radiographs.

- Quality assurance 2 (QA2) Diagnostically acceptable. Some errors present. Patient positioning could be incorrect, exposure time, processing or film handling could be problematic. However, they do not detract from the application of the radiograph and a diagnosis can still be derived. QA2 (Diagnostically acceptable) should be no more than 20%.

- Quality assurance 3 (QA3) Diagnostically unacceptable. Errors present such as patient positioning or tolerance of intraoral film by patient. Exposure time and setting could make film too pale or dark. Processing errors, such as inadequate chemicals in the processing machine or a fault with the digital equipment, can lead to the radiograph being

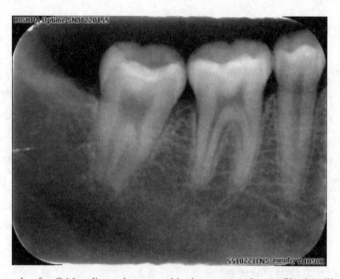

Figure 23.2　Example of a QA1 radiograph: no positioning, processing or film handling errors present.

deemed diagnostically undesirable. QA3 (Diagnostically unacceptable) no more than 10%.

Examples are given in Figures 23.2, 23.3 and 23.4.

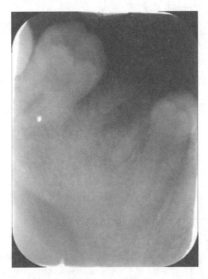

Figure 23.3 Example of a QA2 radiograph: both a positioning error and an exposure time error have occurred but can still be used for diagnostic purposes.

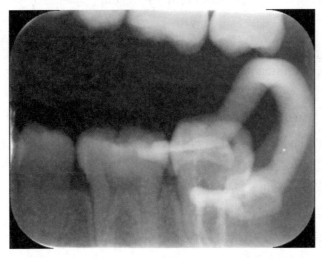

Figure 23.4 Example of a QA3 radiograph: a positioning error has occurred and has rendered this radiograph diagnostically(radiographically) unacceptable.

📝 Word List

1. viewing screen or viewer 观片灯
2. optimal [ˈɒptɪməl] *adj.* 最适宜的；最理想的；最好的
3. uniform [ˈjuːnɪfɔːm] *adj.* 均匀的；一致的；统一的
4. film [fɪlm] *n.* 胶片；影片；膜；胶卷
5. magnifying glass 放大镜
6. contrast [ˈkɒntrɑːst] *n.* 对比(度)；对照；反差；明显的差异
7. facility [fəˈsɪlɪtɪ] *n.* 设施；设备
8. anatomical [ˌænəˈtɒmɪkəl] *adj.* 解剖的；解剖学的
9. foramina [fəˈræmɪnə] *n.* 孔；小孔(foramen 的复数)
10. trabeculae [trəˈbekjələ] *n.* 梁(trabecula 的复数)
11. quality assurance 质量保证
12. ascertain [ˌæsəˈteɪn] *vt.* 确定
13. justification [ˌdʒʌstɪfɪˈkeɪʃn] *n.* 辩解；无过失；正当理由；正当性
14. opacity [əʊˈpæsətɪ] *n.* 不透明性[度]；不反光；混浊度；暗度
15. dental panoramic tomographic (DPT) radiograph 牙科曲面体层片
16. condyle [ˈkɒndɪl] 髁
17. antrum [ˈæntrəm] *n.* 窦(复数形式为 antra)
18. radiopaque [ˌreɪdɪəʊˈpeɪk] *adj.* (X 线，γ 射线等)射线[辐射]透不过的；阻射的
19. obturation material 充填材料
20. radiolucent [ˈreɪdɪəʊˈluːsnt] *adj.* (X 线，γ 射线等)射线可透过的；透射的
21. proximity [prɒkˈsɪmətɪ] *n.* 邻近
22. prescribe [prɪˈskraɪb] *v.* 规定；命令；指示；给……开(药)
23. intraoral film 口内(X 线)胶片
24. exposure time (X 线等)曝光时间；照射时间
25. exposure setting 曝光参数；照射参数(如管电流、管电压等)
26. pale [peɪl] *adj.* 灰白的；苍白的；浅色的

✎ Notes

❶ For digital systems the requirements to view the radiograph are: optimal contrast, brightness and image enhancement, and use of a zoom facility.

对于数字化系统，查看放射影像的要求包括最佳对比度、亮度和锐化度，以及缩放功能的使用。

❷ The World Health Organisation (WHO) has defined radiographic quality assurance (QA) programmes as 'an organized effort by the staff operating a facility to ensure that the diagnostic images produced by the facility are of sufficiently high quality so that they consistently provide adequate diagnostic information at the lowest possible cost and with the least possible exposure of the patient to radiation'.

世界卫生组织(WHO)将放射成像质量保证(QA)方案定义为"由操作设备的工作人员负责实施的一套质量保证操作规程，旨在使设备产生的诊断图像具有足够高的质量，从而持续提供足够的诊断信息，同时以最低的成本和最少的辐射暴露来保护患者"。

❸ Exposure time should be correct for size of patient and position of the tooth/ teeth with no processing or handling faults.

曝光时间应与受检者身材大小、受照牙位置(如上颌或下颌，前牙或后牙)相适应，没有成像胶片(显影和定影)处理错误。

(本单元由程勇选编)

(文字部分选自 *Dentistry at a Glance*, 1st Edition, Part 2, Chapter 12)

Unit 24 ▶ Orthodontic Assessment

1. Orthodontics and Malocclusion

Orthodontics is a specialty of dentistry concerned with facial growth, development of the dentition and occlusion, and the diagnosis, interception, and treatment of occlusal anomalies [1]. 'Ideal occlusion' is the term for a dentition where the teeth are in the optimum anatomical position, both within the upper and lower arches (intramaxillary) and between the arches when the teeth are in occlusion (intermaxillary) [2]. **Malocclusion** means dental anomalies and occlusal traits that represent a deviation from the ideal occlusion.

2. Clinical Assessment in Orthodontics

At the initial orthodontic appointment the following information should be ascertained:

a. What is the complaint?

b. Medical history such as: asthma, epilepsy, diabetes, haemophilia, arthritis, amelogenesis and dentinogensis imperfecta, down syndrome, learning difficulties, temporomandibular joint disorders, nickel allergy and latex allergy.

c. Habits or trauma.

d. Previous orthodontic treatment (may indicate possible compliance issues or an increased risk of root resorption).

本单元正文内容选自 Elizabeth Kay 所著 *Dentistry at a Glance*, John Wiley & Sons, Inc., 2016, Chapter 106, pp.222-223, 选用时删除原文的部分图片, 文字内容有少量改动。

3. Extraoral Examination (Skeletal Assessment)

The patient should be examined sitting upright and focussing on the horizon, with the Frankfort plane (a line joining the inferior margin of the orbit with the superior margin of the external auditory canal) parallel to the floor.

3.1 Anterior-posterior

1. Relationship of soft tissue A and B-point (positions of deepest concavity on maxilla and mandible, respectively):
    a. Skeletal class I: A-point palpable approximately 2 mm ahead of B-point.
    b. Skeletal class II: A-point is palpable >4 mm ahead of B-point
    c. Skeletal class III: B-point is palpable <2 mm behind A-point.
2. Relationship of soft tissue A and B-points to zero-meridian: the zero meridian is represented by a vertical line from the soft tissue nasion (bridge of the nose) perpendicular to the Frankfort plane. Soft tissue A-point should lie on this line and soft tissue B-point should lie approximately 2 mm behind it.

3.2 Vertical

1. The Frankfort-mandibular plane angle (FMPA) should be approximately 27°.
2. Face heights: the middle face height (MFH) and lower face height (LFH) should be equal. MFH is measured from soft tissue glabella to soft tissue subnasale and LFH from subnasale to soft tissue gnathion. LFH is calculated as a percentage of the total face height (TFH = MFH + LAFH) and should be approximately 55%.

3.3 Transverse Assessment

The patient should also be assessed for any facial asymmetry. When an asymmetry is noted, assess for any mandibular displacement on closing, which might be contributing. A compensatory maxillary cant may also be present [3].

4. Soft Tissue Assessment

The following features should be recorded:

1. Lip relationship:
    a. Competent: together at rest.
    b. Potentially competent: able to come together once any dental obstruction has been removed.
    c. Incompetent: apart at rest.
2. Tongue: the tongue is difficult to assess at rest; however, patients that habitually posture the tongue forwards should be noted (can impact on treatment and long-term stability)
3. Nasiolabial angle: the angle formed between the base of the nose and upper lip (94-110°)
4. E-line: a line tangential to the tip of the nose and soft tissue pogonion (should lie ahead of both lips, with the lower lip around 2 mm behind) [4].

5.　Intraoral Examination

Intraoral examination involves: assessment of the teeth present clinically and general dental health (restorations, caries, oral hygiene and periodontal disease).

5.1　For Each Dental Arch

1. Crowding or spacing.
2. Tooth rotations, displacements, impactions.
3. Position and inclination of canines and labial segments to the dental bases.

5.2　In Occlusion

1. Incisor relationship (Figure 24.1)
    a. Class I: the lower incisor edges occlude with or lie below the cingulum plateau of the upper central incisor.
    b. Class II division 1: the lower incisor edges lie posterior to the cingulum plateau of the upper incisors and the upper incisors are proclined/ average inclination and there is an increased overjet.
    c. Class II division 2: the upper incisors are retroclined with a normal or occasionally increased overjet.
    d. Class III: the lower incisor edges lie anterior to the cingulum plateau of the upper incisors.

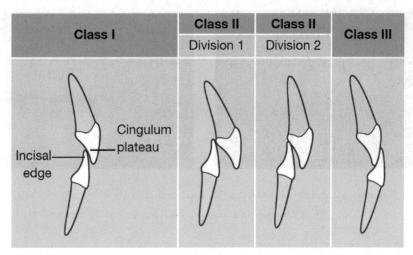

Figure 24.1　Incisor relationship

(选自 *Dentistry at a Glance*, 1st Edition, Part 2, Chapter 106, Figure 106.6)

2. Overjet (measured from most proclined upper incisal edge to the corresponding lower incisor)

3. Overbite (the upper incisors should overlap the lower incisors by a third to half of their clinical crown height)

      a. An increased overbite can be complete to tooth or palate (traumatic when the lower incisors contact the palatal mucosa or the upper incisors contact the lower labial mucosa and cause soft tissue damage (Figure 24.2).

      b. An incomplete overbite is positive overbite with no incisal contact.

      c. An anterior open bite has no vertical overlap between the incisors (Figure 24.2).

4. Molar relationship (Figure 24.3a)

      a. Class I: mesiobuccal cusp of upper first molar occludes with mesiobuccal groove of lower first molar [5].

      b. Class II: mesiobuccal cusp of upper first molar occludes anterior to mesiobuccal groove of lower first molar.

      c. Class III: mesiobuccal cusp of lower first molar occludes mesial to upper first molar mesiobuccal groove.

5. Canine relationship (Figure 24.3b)

6. Centrelines: both should be noted in relation to the facial midline and each other

7. Crossbites: a transverse discrepancy between the dental arches or a premature contact, resulting in a displacement of the mandible on closing.

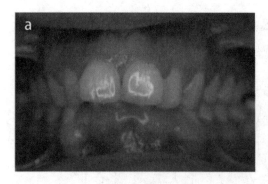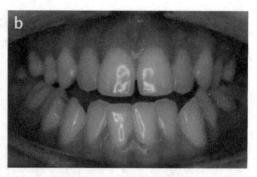

Figure 24.2   Variation in overbite. (a) Increased and complete; (b) open bite.

（选自 *Dentistry at a Glance*, 1st Edition, Part 2, Chapter 106, Figure 106.7)

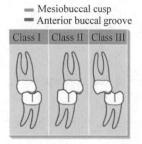

Figure 24.3   (a) Molar relationship; (b) carine relationship.

（选自 *Dentistry at a Glance*, 1st Edition, Part 2, Chapter 106, Figures 106.8 and 106.9）

6. Intraoral Examination

Clinical examination is supplemented by radiographs, study models, extra- and intraoral photographs.

6.1 Radiographic Investigations

a. Dental panoramic tomogram: assess dental development, assessment of unerupted teeth, root morphology, pathology.

b. Lateral cephalogram: assess anterior-posterior and vertical skeletal pattern, incisor inclination and soft tissue profile; can also help with location of unerupted teeth.

c. Upper standard occlusal: diagnose and assess the presence of supernumerary teeth, impacted teeth, root morphology and pathology.

6.2 Study Models

Pretreatment planning, space analysis, treatment progress.

📄 **Word List**

1. orthodontics [ˌɔːθəˈdɒntɪks] *n.* 口腔正畸学
2. crossbite [krɒsˈbaɪt] *n.* 反𬌗
3. overjet [ˈəʊvədʒet] *n.* 覆盖
4. overbite [ˈəʊvəbaɪt] 覆𬌗
5. open bite 开𬌗
6. root resorption 根吸收
7. crowding [ˈkraʊdɪŋ] *n.* 拥挤
8. molar relationship 磨牙关系
9. canine relationship 尖牙关系
10. study model 研究模型
11. lateral cephalogram 头颅侧位片
12. space analysis 间隙分析
13. face height 面高
14. zero-meridian [ˈzɪərəu-məˈrɪdɪən] *n.* 零子午线
15. retroclined [ˈretrouklaɪnd] *adj.* 舌倾的
16. proclined [prəuˈklaɪnd] *adj.* 唇倾的

✎ **Notes**

❶ Orthodontics is a specialty of dentistry concerned with facial growth, development of the dentition and occlusion, and the diagnosis, interception, and treatment of occlusal anomalies.

口腔正畸学是牙医学领域的一个专科，它涉及面部生长和牙列、咬合的发育，以及牙𬌗畸形的诊断、干预与治疗。

❷ 'Ideal occlusion' is the term for a dentition where the teeth are in the optimum anatomical position, both within the upper and lower arches (intramaxillary) and between the arches when the teeth are in occlusion (intermaxillary).

"理想牙合"是指牙列中的牙齿在咬合时，无论从上下颌内部看还是从上下颌之间的关系看，均位于最佳的解剖学位置。

❸ Intraoral examination involves：assessment of the teeth present clinically and general dental health (restorations, caries, oral hygiene and periodontal disease).
口内检查包括对患者现有牙齿的临床检查，以及针对充填体、龋病、口腔卫生、牙周病等口腔健康整体情况的评估。

❹ E-line：a line tangential to the tip of the nose and soft tissue pogonion (should lie ahead of both lips, with the lower lip around 2 mm behind).
E 线：与鼻尖及软组织颏前点相切的一条线，应位于上下唇前方，距离下唇约2mm。

❺ Class Ⅰ molar relationship：mesiobuccal cusp of upper first molar occludes with mesiobuccal groove of lower first molar.
Ⅰ类磨牙关系：上颌第一磨牙的近中颊尖咬合于下颌第一磨牙的近中颊沟内。

（本单元由花放选编）
（文字部分选自 *Dentistry at a Glance*，1st Edition，Part 2，Chapter 106）

Unit 25 ▶ Orthodontic Appliances

1. Fixed Orthodontic Appliances

1.1 Fixed Appliances

Definition: an appliance that is fixed to the teeth by the orthodontist and cannot be removed by the patient.

Mode of action: fixed appliances apply mechanical forces to the teeth in order to achieve a range of tooth movements.

Advantages and disadvantages of fixed appliances are given in Table 25.1.

Table 25.1 Advantages and Disadvantages of Fixed Appliances

Advantage of fixed appliances	Disadvantage of fixed appliances
Multiple tooth movements achievable Controlled root movement in three dimensions	Greater risk of iatrogenic damage (soft tissue trauma, root resorption, decalcification) Susceptible to breakages Plaque control more diffcult

（选自 *Dentistry at a Glance*, 1st Edition, Part 2, Chapter 107, Table 107.1）

Components of a fixed appliance are:

a. Brackets-stainless steel preadjusted edgewise bracket systems are the most common type of fixed appliance

---

本单元正文内容选自 Elizabeth Kay 所著 *Dentistry at a Glance*, John Wiley & Sons, Inc., 2016, Chapters 107 and 108, pp.224-228。

b. Bands and bonded tubes for the molar teeth

c. Archwires, which generate forces that are transmitted to the tooth via the bracket

d. Auxiliaries, which are either attached to or work in conjunction with fixed appliances and help control tooth movement.

1.1.1　Preadjusted Edgewise Brackets

Preadjusted edgewise brackets (Figure 25.1a) have a base, a rectangular edgewise slot for the archwire and a mechanism for holding the archwire in the slot (either tie-wings for an elastomeric ligature or a self-ligating mechanism):

a. Each bracket has a prescription for each individual tooth position built into it.

b. The slot produces mesiodistal tooth angulation or tip.

c. The bracket base inclination provides the necessary torque.

d. The slot to bracket base distance provides the correct on/out position.

There are a variety of bracket variations available:

a. Brackets can be composed of metal (Figure 25.1a), ceramic (Figure 25.1b) or a combination of these materials.

b. Self-ligating brackets engage the archwire using a gate or clip (Figure 25.1c). Self-ligating brackets were introduced in an attempt to reduce friction and clinical time.

c. Lingual brackets are bonded to the lingual and palatal aspects of the teeth and provide optimal aesthetics for the patient (Figure 25.1d); however, they are expensive, clinically challenging and can cause soft tissue irritation of the tongue.

1.1.2　Archwires

The ideal properties of an archwire will depend upon the stage of treatment and type of tooth movement that is being carried out (Table 25.2). Unfortunately, there is no single type of archwire that can be used throughout treatment; instead, a series of different archwires are used as treatment progresses.

Table 25.2　Properties and Applications of Archwires

Archwire material	Archwire properties	Clinical applications
Nickel titanium	Low modulus of elasticity High springback Low continuous force	Excellent aligning archwire, which is able to engage multiple displaced teeth Exerts low forces with little permanent deformation

Continued

Archwire material	Archwire properties	Clinical applications
Stainless steel	Good resistance to deformation Low springback and stored energy Good joinability and formability, therefore you can weld to the archwire and place bends Low friction	Rectangular stainless steel is used for levelling of the occlusal plane, torque expression and space closure Twistflex (multistrand wires) for fixed retainers
Beta-titanium alloy	Properties midway between those of stainless steel and nickel titanium High yield strength Low elastic modulus Medium springback Good formability and weldability	Used as a fnishing archwire as springback allows some deflection of the archwire without permanent deformation. Finishing bends can be placed to detail individual tooth position and achieve occlusal settling
Cobalt chromium	High stiffness Good formability Good biocompatability	Can be hardened by heat-treating in the laboratory and used for the construction of auxiliaries, such as a quadhelix
Aesthetic archwires	Coated archwires are metal with a leflon or epoxy resin coating Poor durability due to failure of the coating and clogging within the bracket slot Composite archwires are constructed from pure silicon dioxide. Poor mechanical properties compared with traditional counterparts	Used when patients request less conspicuous appliances

(选自 *Dentistry at a Glance*, 1st Edition, Part 2, Chapter 107, Table 107.2)

1.1.3   Auxiliaries

a. Separators are used to provide space for band placement on posterior teeth.

b. Elastomeric modules or stainless steel ligatures hold the archwire within the bracket slot.

c. Elastomeric chain can be attached to move single or multiple groups of teeth.

d. Elastic thread can apply traction to individual teeth.

e. Closed or open coil springs can be used to hold, create or close space.

f. Intermaxillary or intramaxillary elastics can be used to translate groups of teeth.

g. Hooks can be attached to the archwire.

Temporary anchorage devices (TADs) are miniscrews inserted intraorally into the bone to provide absolute anchorage [1] (Figure 25.1e).

Headgear consists of a head cap or neck strap attached to a fixed appliance using a Kloehn facebow. The inner part of the bow slots into headgear tubes on molar bands. To reinforce anchorage the headgear is worn for 10-12 hours per day with a force of 250-350 g per side. To distalise the buccal segments and restrain maxillary growth headgear should be worn for longer, up to 14 hours per day with a force of 450-500 g delivered per side.

Transpalatal arches (TPAs) (Figure 25.1f) are constructed of a 0.9-mm stainless steel wire attached to a molar band, which runs across the roof of the mouth. They are used primarily for anchorage reinforcement or the derotation/ expansion of molar teeth.

A quadhelix (Figure 25.1g) is used for maxillary arch expansion and crossbite correction. The appliance sits in the palatal vault and consists of four helices made from 0.9 to 1-mm stainless steel attached to molar bands. The palatal arms apply a lateral force to the buccal segments.

1.2　Stages of Treatment with Fixed Appliances

Treatment with preadjusted edgewise fixed appliances involves a number of stages, including alignment and leveling of the arches, space closure and co-ordination of the arches to achieve a class I incisor relationship [2] (Figure 25.2).

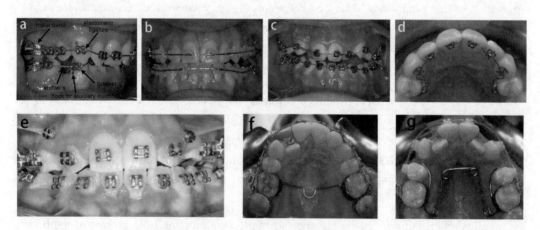

Figure 25.1　(a) Components of a fixed appliance; (b) ceramic preadjusted edgewise brackets; (c) self-ligating preadjusted edgewise brackets; (d) lingual brackets (source: courtesy of Dirk Bister); (e) temporary anchorage device; (f) transpalatal arch; (g) quadhelix.

（选自 *Dentistry at a Glance*, 1st Edition, Part 2, Chapter 107, Figures 107.1 and 107.3-107.8）

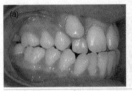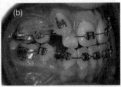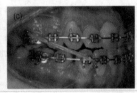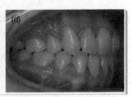

Figure 25.2 Stages of treatment with fixed appliances: (a) treatment of a crowded class III case involved extraction of four first premolars, (b) alignment and leveling, (c) space closure and arch co-ordination to obtain (d) a class I occlusion.

(选自 *Dentistry at a Glance*, 1st Edition, Part 2, Chapter 107, Figure 107.9)

2. Removable Orthodontic Appliances

2.1 Removable Appliances

Definition: Removable appliances can be taken out of the mouth by the patient.

Mode-of-action: Removable appliances apply mechanical forces to the teeth but with a restricted range of movement.

Types of removable appliance are:

　　a. Acrylic.

　　b. Retainers.

　　c. Functional appliances.

　　d. Aligners.

Removable appliances can be used in a number of clinical situations and can achieve:

　　a. Tipping of teeth.

　　b. Correction of anterior or posterior crossbites.

　　c. Overbite reduction.

　　d. Space maintenance.

　　e. Vertical anchorage during the extrusion of unerupted teeth.

　　f. Maxillary protraction or restraint in conjunction with reverse or conventional headgear, respectively.

　　g. Growth modification.

　　h. Alignment of mild crowding.

2.1.1 Acrylic Appliances

Acrylic removable appliances and some retainers are conventionally made of an acrylic base plate, retentive and active components (Tables 25.3-25.5). Clasps are used anteriorly and posteriorly to stabilise a removal appliance.

2.1.2   Retainers

Retainers are appliances designed to maintain the position of the teeth following orthodontic treatment [3] (Table 25.6).

Table 25.3   Acrylic Base Plate

Component	Description
Passive acrylic base plate	Complete palatal coverage and extension ensures no undesired tooth movement and vertical anchorage
Flat anterior bite plane	For reduction of an increased overbite in a growing patient. Separatlon of the posterior occlusion by 1-2 mm, encourages the posterior molars to erupt, reducing the overbite
Inclined anterior bite plane	Can encourage and retain musculoskeletal correction of a skeletal II malocclusion following functional appliance treatment
Posterior bite plane	Used to open the bite during correction of anterior and posterior crossbites
Incorporation of a midline screw	Correction of a buccal crossbite through activation of a midline expansion screw (1 turn per week at 0.25 mm per turn)
Addition of prosthetic teeth	As well as offering an aesthetic solution prosthetic teeth can act as a space maintainer following premature loss of a tooth, particularly an incisor, where they prevent drifing of adjacent teeth, loss of space and maintain the centreline

Table 25.4   Retention

Tooth	Diameter of stainless steel wire (mm)	Name of clasp
654|456	0.7	Adams clasp (first molars and premolars)
6E|E6	0.6	Double Adams crib Useful in the late mixed dentition
4|4	0.7	Adams clasp
1|1	0.7	Southend clasp provides increased anterior retention

Table 25.5 Active Components

Active component	Diameter of stainless steel wire (mm)	Indication and mode of activation
Z-spring (Figure 108.1)	0.5	To move an incisor labially
Double Z-spring	0.6	To move two anterior teeth labially
T-spring	0.6	To move incisors labially and premolars or molars buccally
Cantilever spring	0.6	To procline an incisor
Palatal finger springs	0.5	To move a canine mesially or distally
Buccal canine retractor	0.5 (with sleeve) or 0.7	For retraction of mesially angulated canines
Roberts retractor	0.5 with tubing	Useful for tipping proclined maxillary incisors
Labial bow	0.7	Can be used to retract incisors or simply provide retention

Table 25.6 Retainers

Type of retainer	Mode of action
Hawley retainer	Retained with Adams cribs on the first molars and an anterior labial bow that can have acrylic added (acrylated) to improve retention and prevent rotation
Begg retainer	A horseshoe-shaped labial bow that extends around the dentition allowing occlusal settling
Vacuum-formed retainer	Clear thermoplastic retainers that fit tightly around the entire dentition Aesthetically pleasing and cost effective

(Note：以上 Tables 均选自 *Dentistry at a Glance*，1st Edition，Part 2，Chapter 108，Tables 108.1-108.4)

2.1.3 Functional Appliances

Functional appliances are designed to change the postural position of the mandible in growing patients, with the aim of correcting the functional environment of the dentition and influencing the position of the teeth and growth of the jaws [4]. In class II cases, the aim is to encourage mandibular growth, whilst in class III cases mandibular growth is restrained and maxillary growth encouraged. Functional appliances are used very successfully in the management of class II malocclusions (Figures 25.3 and 25.4).

Functional appliances used to treat a skeletal class II patterns have similar effects:

    a. Retroclination of the upper incisors.

    b. Proclination of the lower incisors.

    c. Distal tipping of the maxillary dentition.

    d. Mesial eruption of the mandibular buccal dentition.

    e. Restraint of maxillary development.

    f. Anterior growth and remodelling of the mandibular condyle and glenoid fossa.

2.1.4 Aligners

Aligners are clear plastic trays that are worn full time by the patient and changed on a regular basis to achieve desired tooth movements [5].

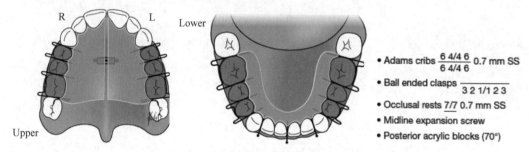

- Adams cribs $\frac{6\ 4/4\ 6}{6\ 4/4\ 6}$ 0.7 mm SS
- Ball ended clasps $\frac{}{3\ 2\ 1/1\ 2\ 3}$
- Occlusal rests 7/7 0.7 mm SS
- Midline expansion screw
- Posterior acrylic blocks (70°)

Figure 25.3   Modified twin block appliance design

(选自 *Dentistry at a Glance*, 1st Edition, Part 2, Chapter 108,Figure 108.3)

2.2 Fitting a Removable Appliance

1. Check the appliance is for the correct patient.
2. Feel the fitting surface of the acrylic base plate for any areas of roughness and smooth if indicated.
3. Show the patient the appliance and explain what the aims are.
4. Try the appliance in and adjust accordingly to ensure optimal retention.
5. Demonstrate the mode of insertion and removal and ensure the patient is competent to carry out this unaided.

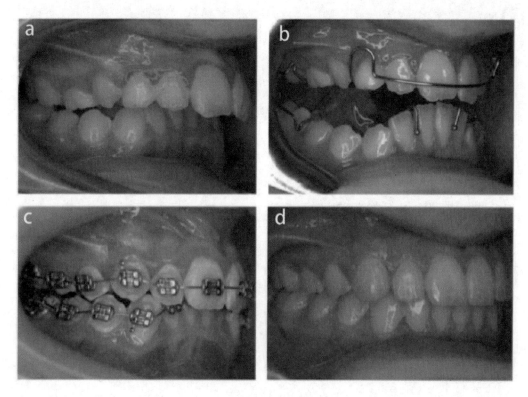

Figure 25.4   Twin block functional appliance and then fixed appliances used to correct a class II division
1 malocclusion

（选自 *Dentistry at a Glance*, 1st Edition, Part 2, Chapter 108, Figure 108.4）

6. Verbal and written instructions for the following should be provided:

    a. Full-time wear.

    b. Remove to clean teeth and appliance.

    c. Remove appliance for sport and wear a gumshield if indicated.

    d. Initially speech will be affected; however, this will improve with time.

    e. Initial wear will result in increased saliva production.

    f. Contact the orthodontist if there is any discomfort, breakage or loss.

7. A review should be made in 2 weeks to ensure adaption and compliance.

8. A review should be made in 4 weeks for re-activation of springs and to assess
treatment progression.

🗏 Word List

1. bracket [ˈbrækɪt] *n.* 托槽
2. self-ligating bracket 自锁托槽
3. temporary anchorage devices（TADs）临时支抗装置
4. transpalatal arch（TPA）横腭杆
5. alignment [əˈlaɪnmənt] *n.* 排齐
6. leveling [ˈlevəlɪŋ] *n.* 整平
7. band [bænd] *n.* 带环 *v.* 粘带环于……
8. preadjusted edgewise fixed appliance 预调方丝弓固定矫治器
9. archwire [ˈɑːtʃwaɪə(r)] *n.* 弓丝
10. torque [tɔː(r)k] *n.* 转矩
11. functional appliance 功能矫治器
12. twin block appliance 双𬌗垫矫治器
13. aligner [əˈlaɪnə(r)] *n.* 无托槽隐形矫治器
14. headgear [ˈhedɡɪə(r)] *n.* 头帽-口外弓；帽子
15. retainer [rɪˈteɪnə(r)] *n.* 保持器
16. vacuum-formed retainer 真空压膜保持器
17. quadhelix [kwɒdˈhiːlɪks] *n.* 四眼圈簧扩弓器

✍ Notes

❶ Temporary anchorage devices（TADs）are miniscrews inserted intraorally into the bone to provide absolute anchorage.

临时支抗装置是口内植入骨中的微螺钉，其目的是提供绝对支抗。

❷ Treatment with preadjusted edgewise fixed appliances involves a number of stages, including alignment and leveling of the arches, space closure and co-ordination of the arches to achieve a class Ⅰ incisor relationship.

采用预调方丝弓固定矫治器进行治疗通常涉及几个步骤，包括排齐整平牙弓、关闭间隙，以及协调上下颌牙弓以达到Ⅰ类切牙关系。

❸ Retainers are appliances designed to maintain the position of the teeth following orthodontic treatment.

保持器是一种矫治器，用于维持正畸治疗后牙齿的位置。

❹ Functional appliances are designed to change the postural position of the mandible in growing patients, with the aim of correcting the functional environment of the dentition and influencing the position of the teeth and growth of the jaws.

功能矫治器用于改变生长发育期患者下颌姿势位，目的是纠正牙列的功能环境，对牙齿位置及颌骨发育施加影响。

❺ Aligners are clear plastic trays that are worn full time by the patient and changed on a regular basis to achieve desired tooth movements.

无托槽隐形矫治器是一种透明塑料托盘，由患者全时戴用，定期更换，以此实现期望达到的牙齿移动。

（本单元由花放选编）

（文字部分选自 *Dentistry at a Glance*, 1st Edition, Part 2, Chapters 107 and 108）

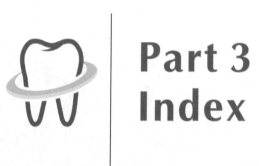

Part 3
Index

Vocabulary

abscess ['æbses] *n.* 脓肿；脓疮   Unit 6

abutment [ə'bʌtmənt] *n.* 基台   Unit 22

accumulation [əˌkjuːmjə'leɪʃn] *n.* 堆积；积聚   Unit 15

acidic [ə'sɪdɪk] *adj.* 酸性的   Unit 14

acidogenic [ˌæsɪdəʊ'dʒenɪk] *adj.* 产酸的   Unit 14

acoustic [ə'kuːstɪk] *adj.* 声音的   Unit 14

acrylic resin 丙烯树脂   Unit 17

actinomyces [ˌæktɪnəʊ'maɪsiːz] *n.* 放线菌属   Unit 5

actinomyces naeslundii 奈瑟氏放线菌   Unit 13

adhesive [əd'hiːsɪv] *adj.* 黏着的；有黏性的 *n.* 黏着剂；胶水 Unit 7

adjunctive [ə'dʒʌŋktɪv] *adj.* 附属的；附加的   Unit 7

adjuncts to biopsy-cytology 辅助活检细胞学检查   Unit 19

adolescent [ˌædə'lesnt] *n.* 青少年   Unit 2

aesthetic [es'θetɪk] *n.* 美学；审美观   Unit 9

aesthetics [es'θetɪks] *n.* 美学   Unit 6

aetiological [iːtɪə'lɒdʒɪkəl] *adj.* 病因论的   Unit 15

aetiology [ˌiːtɪ'ɒlədʒɪ] *n.* [基医]病因学；病原学；原因论 Unit 4

aggregatibacter actinomycetemcomitans 集聚放线菌 Unit 13

aligner [ə'laɪnə] *n.* 无托槽隐形矫治器   Unit 25

219

alignment ［əˈlaɪnmənt］ *n.* 排齐   Unit 25

all-ceramic crown 全瓷冠   Unit 16

alveolar bone 牙槽骨   Unit 12

alveolar crest fibers 牙槽嵴纤维   Unit 12

alveolar ridge 牙槽嵴   Unit 16

amalgam ［əˈmælgəm］ *n.* 汞合金   Unit 6

ameloblastic fibroma 成釉细胞纤维瘤   Unit 21

ameloblastoma ［ˌæməlɒblæsˈtəmə］ *n.* 成釉细胞瘤；造釉细胞瘤；釉母
细胞瘤   Unit 21

amelodentinal junction 釉牙本质界   Unit 9

amine alcohols 氨基醇   Unit 14

amputate ［ˈæmpjuteɪt］ *vt.* 切断   Unit 11

anaerobes ［æˈneərəubz］ *n.* 厌氧菌   Unit 15

anaerobic ［ˌænəˈrəubɪk］ *adj.* 厌氧的   Unit 5

anaesthesia ［ˌænəsˈθiːzɪə］ *n.* 麻醉   Unit 11

anaesthetised ［əˈnesθətaɪzd］ *adj.* 被麻醉的   Unit 10

anatomical ［ˌænəˈtɒmɪkəl］ *adj.* 解剖的；解剖学的   Unit 23

anatomy ［əˈnætəmɪ］ *n.* 解剖；解剖结构   Unit 11

ankylosis ［ˌæŋkɪˈləusɪs］ *n.* ［外科］关节僵硬；胶着   Unit 4

anodontia ［ˌænəˈdɒnʃɪə］ *n.* 无牙；牙缺失   Unit 17

anterior teeth 前牙   Unit 11

antibiotic ［ˌæntɪbaɪˈɒtɪk］ *adj.* 抗生素的   Unit 11

antibiotics ［ˌæntɪbaɪˈɒtɪks］ *n.* 抗生素   Unit 10

antrum ［ˈæntrəm］ *n.* 窦（复数形式为 antra）   Unit 23

apical periodontitis 根尖周炎   Unit 11

appetite ［ˈæpɪtaɪt］ *n.* 胃口；食欲   Unit 6

arch ［ɑːtʃ］ *n.* 牙弓 — Unit 17

archwire ［ˈɑːtʃwaɪə］ *n.* 弓丝 — Unit 25

ascertain ［ˌæsəˈteɪn］ *vt.* 确定 — Unit 23

aspirate ［ˈæspərət］ *v.* 吸气 *n.* 送气音 — Unit 7

aspiration ［ˌæspəˈreɪʃn］ *n.* 抱负；志向；［医］吸引术；抽吸 — Unit 7

asymptomatic ［ˌeɪsɪmptəˈmætɪk］ *adj.* 无症状的 — Unit 21

attachment loss 附着丧失 — Unit 15

attrition ［əˈtrɪʃn］ *n.* 磨损 — Unit 3

axis of rotation 转动轴；支点线 — Unit 17

backfill ［ˈbækfɪl］ *vt.* 回填 — Unit 11

bacterial ［bækˈtɪrɪəl］ *adj.* 细菌的 — Unit 6

band ［bænd］ *n.* 带环 *v.* 粘带环于…… — Unit 25

biofilm ［ˈbaɪəʊfɪlm］ *n.* 生物膜 — Unit 13

biopsy ［ˈbaɪɒpsi］ *n.* 活组织检查；活组织切片检查；切片检查法 — Unit 19

bisbiguanide ［ˌbɪsbɪgwˈɑːnɪd］ *n.* 双胍类化合物 — Unit 14

bracket ［ˈbrækɪt］ *n.* 托槽 — Unit 25

bruit ［bruːt］ *n.* （尤指听诊中听到的）杂音 — Unit 20

buccal ［ˈbʌkəl］ *adj.* （面）颊的 — Unit 11

CAD/CAM 计算机辅助设计/计算机辅助制造 — Unit 16

calcification ［ˌkælsɪfɪˈkeɪʃn］ *n.* 钙化；石灰化 — Unit 21

calcium hydroxide 氢氧化钙 — Unit 10

calculus ［ˈkælkjələs］ *n.* 牙结石 — Unit 12

canine ［ˈkeɪnaɪn］ *n.* 尖牙 — Unit 2

canine relationship 尖牙关系 — Unit 24

cantilever bridge 单端固定桥；悬臂固定桥 — Unit 16

carbohydrate ［ˌkɑːbəʊˈhaɪdreɪt］ *n.* 碳水化合物；糖类 — Unit 5

carboxymethyl ［kɑːbɒkˈsiːmeθɪl］ *n.* 羧甲基　　　　　　　Unit 8

caries risk 龋病风险　　　　　　　Unit 9

caries ［ˈkeəriːz］ *n.* 龋齿　　　　　　　Unit 6

cast ［kɑːst］ *v.* 铸造　　　　　　　Unit 16

cavity ［ˈkævətɪ］ *n.* 窝洞　　　　　　　Unit 9

cellulitis ［ˌseljuˈlaɪtɪs］ *n.* 蜂窝组织炎　　　　　　　Unit 6

cellulose ［ˈseljuləʊs］ *n.* 纤维素　　　　　　　Unit 7

cement ［sɪˈment］ *n.* 水门汀　　　　　　　Unit 16

cementation ［ˌsiːmenˈteɪʃn］ *n.* 黏固；烧结　　　　　　　Unit 7

cementodentinal junction 牙骨质界　　　　　　　Unit 11

cement-retained ［sɪˈment-rɪˈteɪnd］ *adj.* 粘接固位　　　　　　　Unit 22

cementum ［sɪˈmentəm］ *n.* 牙骨质　　　　　　　Unit 12

cetylpyridinium chloride 西吡氯铵　　　　　　　Unit 14

chlorhexidine ［klɔːˈheksɪdaɪn］ *n.* 氯己定；洗必泰　　　　　　　Unit 14

chlorhexidine gluconate 葡萄糖酸氯己定　　　　　　　Unit 14

chronic gingivitis 慢性龈炎　　　　　　　Unit 15

chronological ［ˌkrɒnəˈlɒdʒɪkl］ *adj.* 按时间先后的　　　　　　　Unit 3

clasp ［klɑːsp］ *n.* 卡环　　　　　　　Unit 17

cobalt chromium 钴铬合金　　　　　　　Unit 17

collagen ［ˈkɒlədʒən］ *n.* 胶原蛋白　　　　　　　Unit 12

commence ［kəˈmens］ *vt.* 开始　　　　　　　Unit 2

commensal bacteria 共生细菌　　　　　　　Unit 13

complete denture 全口义齿　　　　　　　Unit 17

compliance ［kəmˈplaɪəns］ *n.* 依从性　　　　　　　Unit 15

compliant ［kəmˈplaɪənt］ *adj.* 顺从的；服从的；符合的；一致的　　　　　　　Unit 10

compomer ［kəmˈpəʊmə］（复合树脂与离子）复合体　　　　　　　Unit 6

composite resin 复合树脂   Unit 9

composite resin strip crowns 复合树脂剥脱冠   Unit 6

comprehensive [ˌkɒmprɪˈhensɪv] *adj.* 综合性的；全面的；有理解力的   Unit 19

concave [kɒnˈkeɪv] *adj.* 凹面的   Unit 14

condenser [kənˈdensə(r)] *n.* 垂直加压器   Unit 11

condyle [ˈkɒndɪl] *n.* 髁   Unit 23

cone [kəʊn] *n.* 圆锥形东西；圆锥体   Unit 11

congenital heart disease 先天性心脏病   Unit 10

congenitally [kənˈdʒenɪtəlɪ] *adv.* 天生地；先天地   Unit 3

connector [kəˈnektə(r)] *n.* 连接体   Unit 16

contamination [kənˌtæmɪˈneɪʃn] *n.* 污染   Unit 7

contemplated [ˈkɒntəmpleɪtɪd] *adj.* 预期的   Unit 18

contouring [kənˈtuərɪŋ] *n.* 轮廓线   Unit 15

contraindication [ˌkɑːntrəˌɪndɪˈkeɪʃn] *n.* 禁忌证   Unit 10

contrast [ˈkɒntrɑːst] *n.* 对比(度)；对照；反差；明显的差异   Unit 23

controllable [kənˈtrəʊləbl] *adj.* 可控制的   Unit 14

coping [ˈkəʊpɪŋ] *n.* 内冠   Unit 16

copious [ˈkəʊpiəs] *adj.* 大量的；丰富的   Unit 11

core [kɔː(r)] *n.* 核   Unit 16

coronal flare 冠状面   Unit 11

cortical [ˈkɔːtɪkəl] *adj.* 皮质的；皮层的；外皮的   Unit 21

cotton wool 药棉   Unit 10

crossbite [krɒsˈbaɪt] *n.* 反𬌗   Unit 24

crowding [ˈkraʊdɪŋ] *n.* 拥挤   Unit 24

crumbly [ˈkrʌmblɪ] *n.* 易碎的   Unit 8

curvature [ˈkɜːvətʃə(r)] *n.* 弯曲；弯曲部分   Unit 11

custom-made cast post 个性化铸造桩   Unit 16

debridement［dɪˈbrɪdmənt］n. 清创术；扩创术   Unit 11

debris［ˈdebriː］n. 残骸；碎屑   Unit 11

deciduous dentition 乳牙列   Unit 2

deciduous teeth（primary teeth）乳牙   Unit 6

definitive crown 最终冠   Unit 16

demineralisation［ˌdemiːnrəlaɪˈzeɪʃən］n. 脱矿   Unit 5

dental amalgam 牙科银汞合金   Unit 9

dental calculus removal 牙结石去除   Unit 13

dental floss 牙线   Unit 14

dental fluorosis 氟牙症   Unit 14

dental panoramic tomographic（DPT）radiograph 牙科曲面体层片   Unit 23

dental tape 洁牙带   Unit 14

dentine［ˈdentiːn］n. 牙质；牙木质   Unit 4

denture base 基托   Unit 17

denture-bearing tissues（DBTs）义齿承托组织   Unit 17

deposition［ˌdepəˈzɪʃn］n. 沉积   Unit 3

deprivation［ˌdeprɪˈveɪʃn］n. 匮乏；剥夺   Unit 15

desensitise［diːˈsensətaɪz］v. 使（病人、神经）对疼痛等无感觉或不敏感   Unit 10

desmoplastic［dezˈmɒplæstɪk］adj. 促结缔组织增生的   Unit 21

desmosome［ˈdesməsəm］n. 桥粒   Unit 12

desquamation［ˌdeskwəˈmeɪʃən］n. 脱落；脱屑   Unit 14

detergent［dɪˈtɜːdʒənt］n. 洗涤剂；去污剂   Unit 14

dexterity［dekˈsterətɪ］n. 灵巧；敏捷   Unit 14

diabetes［ˌdaɪəˈbiːtiːz］n. 糖尿病   Unit 15

dicationic［dɪˈkeɪʃnɪk］adj. 双阳离子的   Unit 14 digital impression 数字化印模   Unit 16

direct retainer 直接固位体   Unit 17

discernible [dɪˈsɜːnəbl] adj. 可识别的；可辨别的   Unit 11

dislodge [dɪsˈlɒdʒ] vt. 把……逐出 vi. 移走；离开原位   Unit 7

dislodgement [dɪsˈlɒdʒmənt] n. 脱位   Unit 17

distolingual [ˌdɪstəʊˈlɪŋgwəl] adj. 远中舌的   Unit 11

divergent [daɪˈvɜːdʒənt] adj. 分散的   Unit 16

dramatically [drəˈmætɪklɪ] adv. 戏剧地；显著地   Unit 7

dynamic [daɪˈnæmɪk] adj. 动态的；发展变化的   Unit 14

dynamic fluid 动态流体   Unit 14

dysbiotic biofilm 失调的生物膜   Unit 15

edentulous [iːˈdentʃələs] adj. 缺齿的；无齿的   Unit 20

edentulousness [iːˈdentʃləsnɪs] n. 无牙颌   Unit 17

electronic apex locator 电子根尖定位仪   Unit 11

elliptical [ɪˈlɪptɪkl] adj. 椭圆的   Unit 19

enamel [ɪˈnæml] n. 搪瓷；珐琅；瓷釉；釉质；指甲油   Unit 4

endodontic files 根管锉   Unit 7

eosinophilic [ˌiəˈsɪnəˈfɪlɪk] adj. 嗜酸性的   Unit 21

epithelial [ˌepɪˈθiːlɪəl] adj. 上皮的   Unit 14

epithelium [ˌepɪˈθiːlɪəm] n. 上皮   Unit 12

equilibrium [ˌiːkwɪˈlɪbrɪəm] n. 平衡   Unit 6

erupt [ɪˈrʌpt] v. 萌出   Unit 6

eruption [ɪˈrʌpʃ(ə)n] n. 萌出   Unit 14

erythematous [ˌerɪˈθiːmətəs] adj. 红斑的   Unit 20

essential oils 精油   Unit 14

etching [ˈetʃɪŋ] n. 蚀刻术；蚀刻版画   Unit 4

ethylene diamine tetracetic acid 乙二胺四乙酸　　　　　　　Unit 11

excavation [ˌekskəˈveɪʃn] v. 挖掘　　　　　　　Unit 8

execute [ˈeksɪkjuːt] v. 执行；实施　　　　　　　Unit 11

exfoliation [eksˌfəʊlɪˈeɪʃn] n. 脱落　　　　　　　Unit 3

exophytic [ˈeksəfaɪtɪk]] adj. 外部生长的　　　　　　　Unit 20

exposure setting 曝光参数；照射参数(如管电流、管电压等)　　　　　　　Unit 23

exposure time(X 线等)曝光时间；照射时间　　　　　　　Unit 23

extracoronal [ˌekstrəˈkɒrəunəl] adj. 冠外的　　　　　　　Unit 16

extraction [ɪkˈstrækʃn] n. (牙齿)拔除；取出　　　　　　　Unit 6

face height 面高　　　　　　　Unit 24

facility [fəˈsɪlətɪ] n. 设施；设备　　　　　　　Unit 23

fermentation [ˌfɜːmenˈteɪʃn] n. 发酵　　　　　　　Unit 6

fibroblast [ˈfaɪbrəblæst] n. 成纤维细胞　　　　　　　Unit 12

file [faɪl] n. 锉；锉刀　　　　　　　Unit 10

film [fɪlm] n. 胶片；影片；膜；胶卷　　　　　　　Unit 23

fissure sealants 窝沟封闭　　　　　　　Unit 6

fixed-fixed bridge 双端固定桥　　　　　　　Unit 16

fixed-movable bridge 固定-活动桥　　　　　　　Unit 16

flange [flændʒ] n. (机械等的)凸缘；(火车的)轮缘　　　　　　　Unit 7

floss [flɒs] n. 牙线 vi. 用牙线清洁牙齿　　　　　　　Unit 7

fluoride [ˈflɔːraɪd] n. 氟化物　　　　　　　Unit 6

foetus [ˈfiːtəs] n. 胎儿　　　　　　　Unit 2

follicular [fəˈlɪkjʊlə] adj. 滤泡的；卵泡的；小囊的　　　　　　　Unit 21

foramina [fəˈræmɪnə] n. 孔；小孔(foramen 的复数)　　　　　　　Unit 23

forceps [ˈfɔːseps] n. 钳子；医用镊子　　　　　　　Unit 18

full crown 全冠　　　　　　　Unit 16

functional appliance 功能矫治器   Unit 25

furcation [fəːˈkeɪʃən] *n.* 分歧；分支   Unit 10

furcation involvement [fəːˈkeɪʃən ɪnˈvɒlvmənt] 分叉病变   Unit 13

fusobacterium nucleatum 核梭杆菌   Unit 13

gauge [geɪdʒ] *n.* 测量的标准或范围；尺度；标准；测量仪器；评估   Unit 7

gauge [geɪdʒ] *n.* 口径；直径   Unit 19

general anaesthesia 全身麻醉   Unit 6

gingiva [dʒɪnˈdʒaɪvə] *n.* 龈   Unit 12

gingival [dʒɪnˈdʒaɪvəl] *adj.* 牙龈的   Unit 7

gingival bleeding 牙龈出血   Unit 14

gingival crevicular fluid（GCF）龈沟液   Unit 13

gingival fibers 牙龈纤维   Unit 13

gingival graft 牙龈移植   Unit 13

gingival margin 龈缘   Unit 13

gingivitis [ˌdʒɪndʒɪˈvaɪtɪs] 龈炎   Unit 12

glass ionomer cement 玻璃离子粘固剂   Unit 9

glass ionomer cements 玻璃离子水门汀   Unit 6

glutamic acid 谷氨酸   Unit 8

glycoprotein [ˌglaɪkəʊˈprəʊtiːn] *n.* 糖蛋白   Unit 5

Gram-negative bacteria 革兰氏阴性菌   Unit 15

Gram-positive bacteria 革兰氏阳性菌   Unit 15

groove [gruːv] *n.* 沟槽   Unit 14

guide plane 导平面   Unit 17

guided tissue regeneration 引导组织再生   Unit 13

gutta percha 牙胶   Unit 11

haemangioma [ˌhɪmændʒɪˈəʊmə] *n.* 血管瘤   Unit 20

haemophilus［ˌhiːməˈfɪləs］*n.* 嗜血杆菌属　　　　　　　　　　Unit 5

haemostasis［hɪˈmɒstəsɪs］*n.* 止血法　　　　　　　　　　　　Unit 18

hamartomas［ˌhæmɑːˈtəʊmə］*n.* 错构瘤　　　　　　　　　　　Unit 21

hamartomatous proliferation of lymphatic vessels 淋巴管错构瘤增生　　Unit 20

handicapped［ˈhændɪkæpt］*adj.* 残疾的　　　　　　　　　　　Unit 14

handpiece［hændˈpiːs］*n.* 牙科手机　　　　　　　　　　　　　Unit 7

headgear［ˈhedɡɪə(r)］*n.* 头帽-口外弓；帽子　　　　　　　　Unit 25

healing cap 愈合基台　　　　　　　　　　　　　　　　　　　Unit 22

hemidesmosome［heˈmaɪdzmʊsəʊm］*n.* 半桥粒　　　　　　　Unit 12

holistic［həʊˈlɪstɪk］*adj.* 整体的；全面的　　　　　　　　　Unit 15

homologous［həˈmɒləɡəs］*adj.* 同源的；类似的　　　　　　　Unit 3

hospitalisation［ˌhɒspɪtələˈzeɪʃn］*n.* 住院治疗　　　　　　Unit 6

hybrid bridge 复合固定桥　　　　　　　　　　　　　　　　Unit 16

hydrostatic［ˌhaɪdrəˈstætɪk］*adj.* 流体静力的　　　　　　Unit 3

hydroxyapatite［ˌhaɪdrɒksɪˈæpətaɪt］*n.*［矿物］羟基磷灰石　Unit 4

hygiene［ˈhaɪdʒiːn］*n.* 卫生；保健　　　　　　　　　　　　Unit 8

hypercementosis［ˌhaɪpəsmenˈtəʊsɪs］*n.* 牙骨质增生　　　Unit 18

hypersensitivity［ˌhaɪpəˌsensəˈtɪvəti］*n.* 高敏感度　　　　Unit 9

hypochlorite［ˌhaɪpəˈklɔːraɪt］*n.* 次氯酸盐　　　　　　　Unit 8

immunosuppressed［ˌɪmjunəʊsəˈprɛst］*adj.* 免疫抑制的　　Unit 10

impede［ɪmˈpiːd］*vt.* 阻碍；妨碍；阻止　　　　　　　　　Unit 11

implant［ɪmˈplɑːnt］*n.* 种植体　　　　　　　　　　　　　Unit 22

implant-retained crown 种植牙冠　　　　　　　　　　　　Unit 16

impression［ɪmˈpreʃən］*n.* 印模　　　　　　　　　　　　Unit 22

impression taking 取模　　　　　　　　　　　　　　　　Unit 7

in situ［ˌɪn ˈsaɪtuː］在原位置；在原处　　　　　　　　　Unit 7

incisor ［ɪnˈsaɪzə(r)］ *n.* 切牙；门牙   Unit 6

indirect pulp capping 间接盖髓术   Unit 10

indirect retainer 间接固位体   Unit 17

individual's caries risk assessment 个性化龋病风险评估   Unit 14

inflammation ［ˌɪnfləˈmeɪʃn］ *n.* 炎症   Unit 14

inhaling ［ɪnˈheɪlɪŋ］ *v.* 吸入(inhale 的现在分词)   Unit 7

interdental brushes 牙间隙刷   Unit 14

interdental cleaning 齿间清洁   Unit 14

interdental papilla 龈乳头   Unit 13

interproximal ［ˌɪntəˈprɒksɪməl］ *adj.* 邻间的   Unit 7

intertubular ［ˌɪntəːˈtjuːbjʊlə］ *adj.* 管间的   Unit 4

intervene ［ˌɪntəˈviːn］ *v.* 干预；干涉   Unit 15

intracoronal ［ˌɪntrəˈkɒrəunəl］ *adj.* 冠内的   Unit 16

intraoperative ［ˌɪntrəˈɒpərətɪv］ *adj.* 手术发生的，术中的   Unit 19

intraoral film 口内(X 线)胶片   Unit 23

intraoral optical scanner 口内光学扫描仪   Unit 16

intraosseous ［ˌɪntrəˈɒsɪəs］ *adj.* 骨内的   Unit 19

inversion ［ɪnˈvɜːʒn］ *n.* 倒置   Unit 7

irreversible pulpitis 不可复性牙髓炎   Unit 10

irritation ［ˌɪrɪˈteɪʃn］ *n.* (身体某部位的)疼痛；刺激(作用)   Unit 7

isolation ［ˌaɪsəˈleɪʃn］ *n.* 隔离；孤立；绝缘   Unit 7

jaw ［dʒɔː］ *n.* 颌；颚   Unit 7

junctional epithelium 结合上皮   Unit 12

justification ［ˌdʒʌstɪfɪˈkeɪʃn］ *n.* 辩解；无过失；正当的理由；正当性   Unit 23

juxtaposition ［ˌdʒʌkstəpəˈzɪʃn］ *n.* 并置；并列；毗邻；并排   Unit 5

keystone microorganism 基石微生物   Unit 13

labial sulcus 唇沟　　　　　　　　　　　　　　　　Unit 7

lactobacilus［ˌlæktəʊbəˈsɪləs］*n.* 乳杆菌属　　　Unit 5

lamina［ˈlæmɪnə］*n.* 叶片；薄层；薄板　　　　　Unit 2

lateral cephalogram 头颅侧位片　　　　　　　　　Unit 24

lateral condensation 侧方加压充填　　　　　　　　Unit 11

latex［ˈleɪteks］*n.* 乳胶；（尤指橡胶树的）橡浆　Unit 7

Ledermix paste 一种由抗生素和类固醇构成的糊剂　Unit 10

leeway space 替牙间隙　　　　　　　　　　　　　Unit 2

leucine［ˈluːsiːn］*n.* 亮氨酸　　　　　　　　　　Unit 8

leucite［ˈluːsaɪt］*n.* 白榴石　　　　　　　　　　Unit 16

leukotoxin［ˌljuːkəʊˈtɒksɪn］*n.* 白细胞毒素　　Unit 13

leveling［ˈlevəlɪŋ］*n.* 整平　　　　　　　　　　Unit 25

leverage force 杠杆力　　　　　　　　　　　　　　Unit 16

ligature［ˈlɪɡətʃə］*n.*（用于紧缚的）带子；绳索；绷带 *v.* 结扎　Unit 7

linger［ˈlɪŋɡə(r)］*v.* 继续存留；缓慢消失；流连；逗留　Unit 10

lingual［ˈlɪŋɡwəl］*adj.* 舌侧的　　　　　　　　　Unit 3

lingual bar 舌杆　　　　　　　　　　　　　　　　Unit 17

lingual plate 舌板　　　　　　　　　　　　　　　Unit 17

lining［ˈlaɪnɪŋ］*n.* 衬层；内衬　　　　　　　　　Unit 10

lipoma［lɪˈpəʊmə］*n.* 脂肪瘤　　　　　　　　　　Unit 19

lobulated［ˈlɒbjʊleɪtɪd］*adj.* 分成小叶的　　　　Unit 20

lymphangioma［lɪmˌfændʒɪˈəʊmə］*n.* 淋巴管瘤　Unit 20

lysine［ˈlaɪsiːn］*n.* 赖氨酸　　　　　　　　　　　Unit 8

magnifying glass 放大镜　　　　　　　　　　　　　Unit 23

maintenance［ˈmeɪntənəns］*n.* 维护；保养　　　Unit 22

major connector *n.* 大连接体　　　　　　　　　　Unit 17

malignancy [məˈlɪɡnənsɪ] *n.* 恶性(肿瘤等)；恶意　　　　Unit 18

malocclusion [ˌmæləˈkluːʒən] *n.* 错牙合畸形　　　　Unit 6

mandatory [ˈmændətərɪ] *adj.* 强制的；命令的　　　　Unit 11

mandible [ˈmændɪbl] *n.* 下颌骨　　　　Unit 2

mandibular [mænˈdɪbjʊlə] *adj.* 下颌的；颚的　　　　Unit 18

manual toothbrushes 手动牙刷　　　　Unit 14

margin [ˈmɑːdʒɪn] *n.* 边缘；边际　　　　Unit 19

marginal ridge 边缘嵴　　　　Unit 10

mastication [ˌmæstɪˈkeɪʃn] *n.* 咀嚼　　　　Unit 6

maxilla [mækˈsɪlə] *n.* 上颌骨　　　　Unit 2

maxillary [mækˈsɪlərɪ] *adj.* 上颌骨的；上颌的 *n.* 上颌骨　　　　Unit 18

maxillary antrum 上颌窦　　　　Unit 18

medically compromised child 医疗条件受限的儿童　　　　Unit 10

medication [ˌmedɪˈkeɪʃn] *n.* 药物；药剂　　　　Unit 11

mesenchyme [ˈmezənkaɪm] *n.* 间质　　　　Unit 21

mesiodistally [ˌmɛsɪə(ʊ)ˈdɪstəlɪ] *adv.* 近远中方向地　　　　Unit 2

metal-ceramic crown 金属烤瓷冠　　　　Unit 16

metallic crown 金属冠　　　　Unit 16

metallic restoration 金属修复材料　　　　Unit 9

microcolony [maɪkˈrɒkələnɪ] *n.* 微小菌落　　　　Unit 15

microorganism [ˌmaɪkrəʊˈɔːɡənɪzəm] *n.* [微]微生物　　　　Unit 7

microporous [ˈmaɪkrəʊˈpɔːrəs] *adj.* 大孔的；大孔隙的；多孔的　　　　Unit 4

mill [mɪl] *v.* 切削；研磨　　　　Unit 16

minor connector 小连接体　　　　Unit 17

mixed dentition 混合牙列　　　　Unit 2

modifiable [ˈmɒdɪfaɪəbl] *adj.* 可修饰的　　　　Unit 15

modified ridge lap pontic 改良盖嵴式桥体　　　　　　　　　　Unit 16

moisture [ˈmɔɪstʃə] *n.* 水分；湿气；潮湿；降雨量　　　　　Unit 7

molar [ˈməʊlə(r)] *n.* 磨牙　　　　　　　　　　　　　　　　Unit 11

molar relationship 磨牙关系　　　　　　　　　　　　　　　　Unit 24

morphogenesis [ˌmɒːfəˈdʒenɪsɪs] *n.* 形态发生　　　　　　Unit 20

morphological [ˌmɔːfəˈlɒdʒɪkl] *adj.* 形态学的　　　　　　Unit 6

morphology [mɔːˈfɒlədʒi] *n.* 形态学　　　　　　　　　　　Unit 2

mouth rinse 漱口水　　　　　　　　　　　　　　　　　　　　Unit 14

mucocele [ˈmjuːkəsiːl] *n.* 黏液囊肿　　　　　　　　　　　Unit 19

mucoperiosteum [ˌmjuːkəʊperɪˈɒstɪəm] *n.* 黏骨膜　　　　Unit 12

mucosa [mjuːˈkəʊsə] *n.* 黏膜　　　　　　　　　　　　　　Unit 14

mucosal support 黏膜支持　　　　　　　　　　　　　　　　Unit 17

mucositis [ˈmjuːkɒsaɪtɪs] *n.* 黏膜炎　　　　　　　　　　Unit 14

multidisciplinary [ˌmʌltɪdɪsəˈplɪnərɪ] *adj.* 多学科的　　Unit 14

multifactorial [ˌmʌltɪfækˈtɒːrɪəl] *adj.* 多因素的　　　　Unit 14

multilocular [ˌmʌltɪˈlɒkjʊlə] *adj.* 多室的；多腔的　　　　Unit 20

muscle balance（MB）肌肉平衡　　　　　　　　　　　　　Unit 17

mutants streptococci 变异链球菌　　　　　　　　　　　　　Unit 5

nasolabial angle 鼻唇角　　　　　　　　　　　　　　　　　Unit 17

necrosis [neˈkrəʊsɪs] *n.* 坏死　　　　　　　　　　　　　Unit 11

negligible [ˈneglɪdʒəbl] *adj.* 可忽略不计的　　　　　　　Unit 15

neoplasm [ˈn(iː)əʊplæzm] *n.* 赘生物；瘤；新生物　　　　Unit 21

neurofibroma [ˌnjʊərəʊfaɪˈbrəʊmə] *n.* 神经纤维瘤　　　Unit 20

nodular [ˈnɒdjʊlə] *adj.* 结节状的；有结节的　　　　　　　Unit 19

normoglycemia [ˌnɔːməʊglaɪˈsiːmɪə] *n.* 血糖正常　　　Unit 15

nutritional deficiency 营养不良　　　　　　　　　　　　　　Unit 15

obesity [əʊˈbiːsəti] *n.* 过度肥胖；肥胖症   Unit 15

obturation material 充填材料   Unit 23

occlusal [əˈkluːs(ə)l] *adj.* 咬合面的   Unit 7

occlusal balance（OB）*n.* 咬合平衡   Unit 17

occlusal contact 咬合接触   Unit 3

occlusal forces 咬合力   Unit 3

occlusal loading 咬合负荷   Unit 16

occlusal plane 咬合面   Unit 2

occlusal registration 咬合记录   Unit 17

occlusal splint 咬合夹板   Unit 17

occlusal trauma 咬合创伤   Unit 13

occlusal wear 咬合磨损   Unit 2

odontoma [ˌɒdɒnˈtəmə] *n.* 牙瘤   Unit 21

oestrogen [ˈiːstrədʒən] *n.* 雌激素   Unit 20

opacity [əʊˈpæsəti] *n.* 不透明性[度]；不反光；混浊度；暗度   Unit 23

open bite 开殆   Unit 24

opposing teeth 对颌牙   Unit 2

optimal [ˈɒptɪməl] *adj.* 最适宜的；最理想的；最好的   Unit 23

oral hygiene measure 口腔卫生措施   Unit 15

oral hygiene 口腔卫生   Unit 10

orthodontic [ˌɔːθəˈdɒntɪk] *adj.* 正畸的；牙齿矫正的   Unit 14

orthodontic [ˌɔːθəˈdɒntɪk] *n.* 口腔正畸术；牙齿矫正   Unit 18

orthodontics [ˌɔːθəˈdɒntɪks] *n.* 口腔正畸学   Unit 24

oscillating [ˌɒsɪˈleɪtɪŋ] *adj.* 振荡的   Unit 14

osseous surgery 骨手术   Unit 13

osseointegration [ˌɒsiːəʊɪntɪɡˈreɪʃn] 骨整合   Unit 22 otitis media 中耳炎   Unit 6

ovate pontic 卵圆形桥体   Unit 16

overbite [ˈəʊvəbaɪt] n. 覆𬌗   Unit 24

overjet [ˈəʊvədʒet] n. 覆盖   Unit 24

oxygenating [ˈɒksɪdʒəneɪtɪŋ] v. 给……供氧   Unit 14

palatal [ˈpælətl] adj. 腭的   Unit 11

pale [peɪl] adj. 灰白的；苍白的；浅色的   Unit 23

papilla gingiva 牙龈乳头   Unit 14

papilloma [ˌpæpɪˈləʊmə] n. 乳头状瘤   Unit 20

parotid duct 腮腺导管   Unit 7

partial crown 部分冠   Unit 16

partial dentures 局部义齿   Unit 15

paste [peɪst] n. 糊剂   Unit 11

pathogenesis [ˌpæθəˈdʒenɪsɪs] n. 发病机理   Unit 15

pathological [ˌpæθəˈlɒdʒɪkl] adj. 病理学的；病态的；由疾病引起的   Unit 18

pellicle [ˈpelɪkl] n. 薄膜   Unit 13

periapical abscess 根尖脓肿   Unit 13

periodontal abscess 牙周脓肿   Unit 13

periodontal charting 牙周记录   Unit 13

periodontal dressing 牙周敷料   Unit 13

periodontal ligament 牙周膜；牙周膜韧带   Unit 3

periodontal maintenance 牙周维护   Unit 13

periodontal pocket 牙周袋   Unit 12

periodontal probe 牙周探针   Unit 12

periodontitis [ˌperɪədɒnˈtaɪtɪs] n. 牙周炎   Unit 12

periodontium [ˌperɪəˈdɒnʃɪəm] n. 牙周组织   Unit 15 periodontopathic [ˌperɪədɒntəˈpæθɪk] *adj.* 导致牙周疾病的　　　Unit 15

periosteal [ˌperɪˈɒstɪəl] *adj.* 骨膜的　　　Unit 18

peripheral seal 边缘封闭　　　Unit 17

periphery [pəˈrɪfərɪ] *n.* 外围；边缘　　　Unit 19

permanent dentition 恒牙列　　　Unit 3

permanent teeth 恒牙　　　Unit 6

pertinent [ˈpɜːtɪnənt] *adj.* 切题的；相关的　　　Unit 19

phenolic compounds 酚类化合物　　　Unit 14

phosphoprotein [fɒsfəʊˈprəʊtiːn] *n.* 磷蛋白　　　Unit 5

physical retention 机械固位　　　Unit 9

pier abutment 中间基牙　　　Unit 16

plaque [plæk] 牙菌斑　　　Unit 6

plaque control 牙菌斑控制　　　Unit 13

plexiform [ˈpleksɪfɔːm] *adj.* (血管等)丛状的　　　Unit 21

polyhedral [ˌpɒlɪˈhiːdrəl] *adj.* 多面的；多面体的　　　Unit 21

polymorphonuclear leukocytes (PMN) 多形核白细胞　　　Unit 13

polyp [ˈpɒlɪp] *n.* 息肉　　　Unit 19

polyvinyl methyl ethyl maleic acid 聚乙烯甲基乙基马来酸　　　Unit 14

pontic [ˈpɒntɪk] *n.* 桥体　　　Unit 16

porcelain [ˈpɔːsəlɪn] *n.* 瓷 *adj.* 瓷制的　　　Unit 16

porosity [pɔːˈrɒsətɪ] *n.* 多孔性　　　Unit 5

porphyromonas gingivalis 牙龈卟啉单胞菌　　　Unit 13

posterior teeth 后牙　　　Unit 11

post-retained crown 桩冠　　　Unit 16

powered irrigation devices 动力灌洗装置　　　Unit 14

powered toothbrushes 电动牙刷　　　Unit 14

preadjusted edgewise fixed appliance 预调方丝弓固定矫治器　　Unit 25

precancerous［ˌpriːˈkænsərəs］癌症前期的　　Unit 19

precision attachment 精密附着体　　Unit 17

predecessor［ˈpredəsesə］n. 前身；（被取代的）原有事物　　Unit 6

predilection［ˌpriːdɪˈlekʃn］n. 偏爱；嗜好　　Unit 20

predominately［prɪˈdɒmɪnətlɪ］adv. 占优势地　　Unit 15

prefabricated［priːˈfæbrɪkeɪtɪd］adj. 预制的　　Unit 16

pregnancy［ˈpregnənsɪ］n. 孕期；妊娠期　　Unit 6

premature loss（牙齿）早失　　Unit 6

preoperative［prɪˈɒpərətɪv］adj. 外科手术前的　　Unit 18

prescribe［prɪˈskraɪb］v. 规定；命令；指示；给……开(药)　　Unit 23

pressed ceramic 铸瓷　　Unit 16

primary dentition 乳牙列　　Unit 3

primary impression 初印模　　Unit 17

primary stability 初期稳定性　　Unit 22

primate spaces 灵长类间隙　　Unit 2

probing depth 探诊深度　　Unit 13

proclined［prəʊˈklaɪnd］adj. 唇倾的　　Unit 24

prophylactic［ˌprɒfəˈlæktɪk］adj. 预防性的；预防疾病的　　Unit 18

prophylaxis［ˌprɒfəˈlæksɪs］n. 预防性清洁术　　Unit 14

proprioception［ˌprəʊprɪəˈsepʃən］n. 本体感受　　Unit 17

proprioceptive［ˌprəʊprɪəˈseptɪv］adj. 本体感受的　　Unit 12

provisional restorations 临时修复体　　Unit 22

proximity［prɒkˈsɪmətɪ］n. 邻近　　Unit 23

public health funding 公共卫生资金　　Unit 15

pulp chamber 髓腔；髓室　　Unit 11

pulp necrosis 牙髓坏死 　　　　　　　　　　　　　　　　　Unit 10

pulpal [ˈpʌlp(ə)l] *adj.* 牙髓的　　　　　　　　　　　　　Unit 7

pulpectomy [pʌlˈpektəmɪ] *n.* 去髓术；牙髓摘除术　　　　Unit 6

pulpotomy [pʌlˈpɔtəmɪ] *n.* 牙髓切断术　　　　　　　　　Unit 6

put... at the risk of 把……置于风险中　　　　　　　　　　Unit 7

pyogenic granuloma 化脓性肉芽肿　　　　　　　　　　　　Unit 20

quadhelix [kwɒdˈhiːlɪks] *n.* 四眼圈簧扩弓器　　　　　　Unit 25

quadrant [ˈkwɔdrənt] *n.* 四分之一圆　　　　　　　　　　Unit 7

quality assurance 质量保证　　　　　　　　　　　　　　　Unit 23

quaternary ammonium compounds 季铵类化合物　　　　Unit 14

radicular [ræˈdɪkjʊlə(r)] *adj.* 根的；小根的　　　　　　Unit 4

radiograph [ˈreɪdɪəʊˌɡræf] *n.* 射线照片 *vt.* [核]拍射线照片　Unit 10

radiolucency [ˌreɪdɪəʊˈljuːsənsɪ] *n.* 射线透射性；射线可透性　Unit 10

radiolucent [ˌreɪdɪəʊˈluːsnt] *adj.* (X线；γ射线等)射线可透过的；透射的　Unit 23

radiopaque [ˌreɪdɪəʊˈpeɪk] *adj.* (X线；γ射线等)射线[辐射]透不过的；阻射的　Unit 23

reamer [ˈriːmə] *n.* [机]铰刀；钻孔器　　　　　　　　　Unit 7

recapitulate [riːkəˈpɪtʃuleɪt] *v.* 重述；概括　　　　　Unit 11

recline [rɪˈklaɪn] *v.* 斜倚　　　　　　　　　　　　　Unit 18

remineralization [ˌremiːnrəlaɪˈzeɪʃn] *n.* 再矿化；未矿化作用　Unit 5

removable partial denture (RPD) 可摘局部义齿　　　　Unit 17

resin-bonded bridge 树脂粘接桥　　　　　　　　　　　Unit 16

rest [rest] *n.* 支托　　　　　　　　　　　　　　　　Unit 17

restoration [ˌrestəˈreɪʃn] *n.* 修复体　　　　　　　　　Unit 16

restorative [rɪˈstɔːrətɪv] *adj.* 整形的；修复性的　　　Unit 6

restorative dentistry［医］牙科修复学　　　　　　　　　　　　Unit 7

retainer［rɪˈteɪnə(r)］n. 保持器　　　　　　　　　　　　　　Unit 25

retainer［rɪˈteɪnə(r)］n. 固位体　　　　　　　　　　　　　　Unit 16

retention［rɪˈtenʃn］n. 固位　　　　　　　　　　　　　　　Unit 17

retract［rɪˈtrækt］vt. & vi. 撤回或撤消；缩回；缩进　　　　　Unit 7

retrieval［rɪˈtriːvl］n. 收回；挽回；检索　　　　　　　　　Unit 7

retroclined［ˈretrouklaɪnd］adj. 舌倾的　　　　　　　　　　Unit 24

retruded contact position（RCP）后退接触位　　　　　　　　Unit 17

reversible pulpitis 可复性牙髓炎　　　　　　　　　　　　　Unit 10

ridge lap pontic 盖嵴式桥体　　　　　　　　　　　　　　　Unit 16

rinse［rɪns］vt. 漂洗；冲洗；漂净　　　　　　　　　　　　Unit 11

root canal orifice 根管口　　　　　　　　　　　　　　　　Unit 11

root canal 根管　　　　　　　　　　　　　　　　　　　　Unit 10

root resorption 根吸收　　　　　　　　　　　　　　　　　Unit 24

rotating［rəʊˈteɪtɪŋ］adj. 旋转的　　　　　　　　　　　　Unit 14

rubber dam clamp 橡皮障夹　　　　　　　　　　　　　　　Unit 7

rubber dam punch 橡皮障打孔器　　　　　　　　　　　　　Unit 7

rubber dam 橡皮障　　　　　　　　　　　　　　　　　　　Unit 7

saddle［ˈsædl］n. 鞍基　　　　　　　　　　　　　　　　　Unit 17

saliva ejector 吸唾器　　　　　　　　　　　　　　　　　　Unit 7

salivary gland 唾液腺　　　　　　　　　　　　　　　　　　Unit 14

sanitary pontic 卫生桥体；悬空式桥体　　　　　　　　　　Unit 16

scaling and root planing 刮治和根面平整　　　　　　　　　Unit 13

sclerosis［skləˈrəʊsɪs］n. 硬化；硬化症；细胞壁硬化　　　　Unit 18

screw-retained［ˌskruː-rɪˈteɪnd］adj. 螺丝固位　　　　　　Unit 22

seal［siːl］v. 封上；密封 n. 印章；图章；密封物　　　　　Unit 10

sealant ［ˈsiːlənt］ *n.* 封闭剂   Unit 14

sealer ［ˈsiːlə(r)］ *n.* 封闭剂   Unit 11

secondary dentin 继发性牙本质   Unit 10

selective grinding 选磨   Unit 17

self-ligating bracket 自锁托槽   Unit 25

self-threading ［selfˈθredɪŋ］ *adj.* 自攻螺纹的   Unit 16

semipermeable ［ˈsemɪˈpɜːmɪəbl］ *adj.* 半渗透的   Unit 4

sequelae ［sɪˈkwiːliː］ *n.* 并发症(sequela 的复数)；后遗症   Unit 6

Sharpey fibers 夏比纤维   Unit 12

sinus ［ˈsaɪnəs］ *n.* 窦道   Unit 10

social inequalities 社会不平等   Unit 15

sodium chlorite 次氯酸钠   Unit 14

sonic ［ˈsɒnɪk］ *adj.* 声波的   Unit 14

space analysis 间隙分析   Unit 24

space maintainers 间隙保持器   Unit 6

spirochaete ［ˈspaɪərəkiːt］ *n.* 螺旋体   Unit 13

spirochaetes ［spɪərəˈtʃiːts］ *n.* 螺旋体   Unit 15

spontaneously ［spɒnˈteɪnɪəslɪ］ ad*v.* 自发地；不由自主地；自然地   Unit 20

spreader ［ˈspredə(r)］ *n.* 侧压器   Unit 11

stability ［stəˈbɪlətɪ］ *n.* 稳定   Unit 17

stainless steel crowns 不锈钢金属冠(金属预成冠)   Unit 6

stannous fluoride 氟化亚锡   Unit 14

stellate ［ˈsteleɪt］ *adj.* 星形的；似星的；放射线状的   Unit 21

streptococcus ［ˌstreptəˈkɒkəs］ *n.* 链球菌属   Unit 5

stretched to 拉伸到   Unit 7

study model 研究模型   Unit 24

subgingival [ˌsʌbdʒɪnˈdʒaɪvəl] *adj.* 龈下的   Unit 13

subgingival plaque 龈下菌斑   Unit 15

suborbital [sʌbˈɔːbɪtəl] *adj.* 眶下的   Unit 6

suction [ˈsʌkʃn] *n.* 吸；抽吸；吸出；相吸   Unit 7

sulcus [ˈsʌlkəs] *n.* 沟；槽；裂缝   Unit 7

supernumerary [ˌsuːpəˈnjuːmərərɪ] *n.* 多生牙；*adj.* 多余的；过剩的   Unit 2

support [səˈpɔːt] *n.* 支持   Unit 17

supportive periodontal care regime 支持性牙周护理方案   Unit 15

supragingival calculus 龈上结石   Unit 14

surgical stent 手术导板   Unit 22

surveyed crown 观测线冠   Unit 16

surveying line 观测线   Unit 17

susceptible [səˈseptəbl] *adj.* 易感的   Unit 6

swelling [ˈswelɪŋ] *n.* 肿块；肿胀处   Unit 10

symptomatic [ˌsɪmptəˈmætɪk] *adj.* 有症状的；症候的   Unit 18

syringe [sɪˈrɪndʒ] *n.* 注射器；注射筒；灌肠器；注油筒；洗涤器   Unit 7

tactile [ˈtæktaɪl] *adj.* 触觉的；能触知的；有形的   Unit 11

tannerella forsythia 福赛氏坦纳菌   Unit 13

temporary anchorage devices（TADs）临时支抗装置   Unit 25

temporary crown 暂时冠   Unit 16

temporomandibular joint（TMJ）颞下颌关节   Unit 18

tertiary [ˈtɜːʃəri] *adj.* 第三的；第三位的；第三级的   Unit 4

tooth mobility 牙齿松动   Unit 13

tooth preparation 牙体预备   Unit 16

tooth support 牙支持   Unit 17

toothpick [ˈtuːθpɪk] *n.* 牙签   Unit 14 topical ['tɒpɪkl] *adj.* 局部的   Unit 14

torque [tɔː(r)k] *n.* 转矩   Unit 25

torquing force 扭力   Unit 16

trabeculae [trə'bekjələ] *n.* 梁(trabecula 的复数)   Unit 23

transpalatal arch (TPA) 横腭杆   Unit 25

trauma ['trɔːmə] 挫折；精神创伤；心理创伤；损伤；外伤   Unit 18

traumatic neuroma 创伤性神经瘤   Unit 20

treponema denticola 齿垢螺旋体   Unit 13

trigeminal [traɪ'dʒemɪnl] *adj.* 三叉神经的   Unit 20

tungsten ['tʌŋstən] *n.* 钨   Unit 8

twin block appliance *n.* 双牙合垫矫治器   Unit 25

ubiquitous [juː'bɪkwɪtəs] *adj.* 无处不在的；普遍存在的   Unit 2

ugly duckling stage 丑小鸭时期   Unit 2

unaesthetic [ˌʌniːs'θetɪk] *adj.* 无美感的   Unit 14

undercut [ˌʌndə'kʌt] *n.* 倒凹   Unit 9

underpin [ˌʌndə'pɪn] *v.* 支撑；加强；构成   Unit 8

uniform ['juːnɪfɔːm] *adj.* 均匀的；一致的；统一的   Unit 23

unilocular [ˌjuːnɪ'lɒkjʊlə] *adj.* 单室的；单房的   Unit 21

vacuum-formed retainer 真空压膜保持器   Unit 25

vascular malformation 脉管畸形   Unit 20

vertical condensation 垂直加压充填   Unit 11

vibration [vaɪ'breɪʃn] *n.* 震动；颤动   Unit 14

viewing screen or viewer 观片灯   Unit 23

viscosity [vɪ'skɒsəti] *n.* 黏性；黏度；黏滞物   Unit 3

vital pulpotomy 活髓切断术   Unit 10

waxed floss [医]有蜡牙线   Unit 7

wax-up ['wæks-ʌp] *n.* 蜡型   Unit 22

xylitol ['zaɪlɪtɒl] *n.* 木糖醇   Unit 14

zero-meridian ['zɪərəu-mə'rɪdɪən] *n.* 零子午线   Unit 24

zinc citrate 柠檬酸锌   Unit 14

zinc oxide cement 氧化锌水门汀   Unit 10

zirconia [zə'kəunɪə] *n.* 氧化锆   Unit 16